Women's Health

D0511844

A practical guide for healthcare professionals

WITHDRAWN

Sarah Bekaert

Advanced Nurse Practitioner
City and Hackney Teaching Primary Care Trust, London

Radcliffe Publishing
Oxford • New York

40p

Radcliffe Publishing Ltd
18 Marcham Road
Abingdon
Oxon OX14 1AA
United Kingdom

www.radcliffe-oxford.com
Electronic catalogue and worldwide online ordering facility.

© 2007 Sarah Bekaert

Sarah Bekaert has asserted her right under the Copyright, Designs and Patents Act 1998 to be identified as author of this Work.

All rights reserved. No part of this publication may be reproduced, stored in a retrieval system or transmitted, in any form or by any means, electronic, mechanical, photocopying, recording or otherwise without the prior permission of the copyright owner.

British Library Cataloguing in Publication Data

A catalogue record for this book is available from the British Library.

ISBN-13: 978 1 84619 029 2

Typeset by Aarontype Ltd, Easton, Bristol
Printed and bound by TJ International Ltd, Padstow, Cornwall

Contents

Preface

The idea of writing this guide arose from working in an acute and community setting in women's health. With the primary focus on sexual health and contraception, the concerns presented by patients often fall into the arenas of gynaecology, early pregnancy and general health. Although working relationships across these areas are good, and specialist practitioners are keen to support each other and to facilitate the patient journey, they are not always immediately available at the end of the phone. This book aims to offer the practitioner a quick reference guide to the possible diagnoses according to symptoms, and the tests that could be performed with a view to reaching a diagnosis. In order to provide a comprehensive guide, brief descriptions of conditions and tests are included. As well as informing the practitioner, this will facilitate information giving to the patient. I have also included sections on contraception and sexual health, as certainly for a significant proportion of many women's lives, the control or facilitation of their reproductive ability is a primary focus.

Sarah Bekaert
June 2007

About the author

Sarah Bekaert is Advanced Nurse Practitioner for City and Hackney Teaching Primary Care Trust, London. She gained her first degree in French studies at Manchester University, and subsequently worked for the relief and development agency Tearfund. She then trained as a paediatric nurse at City University, and has worked in paediatrics, school nursing, practice nursing, a development nurse for Hackney's young people's sexual health services and Senior Practitioner at the Margaret Pyke Centre. Since qualifying she has obtained an MSc in Gynaecology and Reproductive Health Care at Warwick University. She is an associate member of the Faculty of Family Planning and Reproductive Health Care, and a member of the British Association for Sexual Health and HIV and an assessor for the Royal College of Nursing distance learning course in sexual health skills.

List of abbreviations

ACTH	adrenocorticotropic hormone
AIDS	acquired immunodeficiency syndrome
APTT	activated partial thromboplastin time
βHCG	beta human chorionic gonadotropin
BMI	body mass index
BV	bacterial vaginosis
CAH	congenital adrenal hyperplasia
CIN	cervical intra-epithelial neoplasia
CNS	central nervous system
COC	combined oral contraceptive
CRP	C-reactive protein
CS	Caesarean section
CT	computerised tomography
D&C	dilation and curettage
DCIS	ductal carcinoma *in situ*
ERPC	evacuation of retained products of conception
ESR	erythrocyte sedimentation rate
FBC	full blood count
FNA	fine-needle aspiration
FSH	follicle-stimulating hormone
GnRH	gonadotropin-releasing hormone
GUTB	genito-urinary tuberculosis
HCG	human chorionic gonadotropin
HIV	human immunodeficiency virus
HPV	human papilloma virus
HRT	hormone replacement therapy
HSV	herpes simplex virus
ICSI	intracytoplasmic sperm injection
IDDM	insulin-dependent diabetes mellitus
IM	intramuscular
IUD	intrauterine device
IUFD	intrauterine fetal death
IUI	intrauterine insemination
IV	intravenous
IVF	*in-vitro* fertilisation
LCIS	lobular carcinoma *in situ*
LFTs	liver function tests
LH	luteinising hormone
LMP	last menstrual period
LOD	laparoscopic ovarian diathermy

MC&S	microscopy, culture and sensitivity
MCH	mean corpuscular haemoglobin
MCV	mean corpuscular volume
MPV	mean platelet volume
MRI	magnetic resonance imaging
MSU	midstream urine
NSAIDs	non-steroidal anti-inflammatory drugs
PCB	post-coital bleeding
PCV	packed cell volume
PCOS	polycystic ovarian syndrome
PID	pelvic inflammatory disease
PMDD	premenstrual dysphoric disorder
PMS	premenstrual syndrome
PT	prothrombin time
PTT	partial thromboplastin time
PV	per vagina
RBC	red blood cell
STI	sexually transmitted infection
TB	tuberculosis
TFTs	thyroid function tests
TRH	thyrotropin-releasing hormone
TSH	thyroid-stimulating hormone
TV	*Trichomonas vaginalis*
U&Es	urea and electrolytes
USS	ultrasound scan
UTI	urinary tract infection
VIN	vulval intra-epithelial neoplasia
WBC	white blood cell; white blood count

Introduction

This book has come about through my work as a nurse specialist in women's health in various settings, including community contraception clinics, a hospital-based sexual health clinic and an early pregnancy advisory unit in an inner-city multicultural community. During my years in this role I have found many common themes among the symptoms with which women present across these areas. I feel that these themes could usefully be brought together for other clinicians working in similar or related areas.

Despite major scientific advances, women's health needs are still mainly focused around their unique reproductive role, including contraception, unplanned pregnancy, pregnancy, infertility, loss of fertility, body image and self-esteem. I wanted to bring together information that could be used across these and other settings in which women seek health advice (e.g. general practice, Accident and Emergency departments) in a simple quick-reference format.

This book aims to aid the clinician in making a diagnosis via the 'symptom sorter' format, and to provide information about the possible diagnoses and investigations that may be required. When one first meets a patient, they may present with one or a series of symptoms, and the healthcare professional begins the process of reaching a diagnosis – by taking a history and performing an examination and investigations. This book is designed to be used as an on-the-spot quick reference in clinic to guide the clinician's thought processes in eliciting a possible diagnosis, while also providing basic information on conditions, tests required and links to useful related resources.

In order to maintain a patient-focused approach, I have chosen to present the book in the way that a patient would approach their complaint:

- This is my complaint. What could it be? *Symptom sorter.*
- Could you give me more information about the conditions that I might have? *Basic information about possible diagnoses.*
- What tests are involved in finding out what the condition could be, or eliminating certain possibilities? *An explanation of the most common tests and procedures.*
- Where can I find out more about these conditions? *Reputable resources to support information given in the consultation.*

The language used is also patient focused, and uses the vernacular to facilitate understanding. Indeed the layperson would find this book useful for exploring women's health concerns.

I have included the most common symptoms with which patients present in the community and acute sector. The list is not exhaustive, but may offer guidance for a similar symptom. More often than not, certain conditions present with several symptoms, and looking up all symptoms can elicit a common diagnosis. To maximise ease of use, the differential diagnoses exclude extremely rare conditions. It would be hoped that in such cases the healthcare professional would seek specialist advice.

It is recognised that books quickly date, and for the safety of their patients, clinicians are required to use up-to-date evidence-based care. Therefore it is important to update their knowledge through journals, forums and, of course, reliable Internet resources. In view of this I have included signposts to resources that can offer the reader the latest information on a particular subject area.

Format

My inspiration for this format is the excellent book by Hopcroft and Forte entitled *Symptom Sorter* (third edition, also published by Radcliffe), which covers general symptoms. The present book focuses specifically on women's health issues.

Symptom sorter

I have attempted to group symptoms under the common headings of menstrual symptoms, hormonal changes, sexual health, breast symptoms, urinary symptoms, pregnancy and weight, and under these headings symptoms are listed in alphabetical order. However, it is important to be aware that a symptom which may appear to fall within one category can turn out, unexpectedly, to be from another.

Overview

For each symptom I have attempted to give an overview, including the prevalence of the symptom, the age group of women it usually affects, the possible seriousness of the complaint, and any other useful relevant information.

History

An accurate diagnosis always hinges on a comprehensive and relevant history, so I have included specific areas for consideration within a general history in relation to specific symptoms.

Differential diagnosis/possible investigations

The differential diagnosis categorises diagnoses as common, occasional or rare in terms of occurrence. Possible tests and investigations are listed in order from basic to more invasive ones that may be required to aid diagnosis.

Notes

Finally, where appropriate in this initial section, tips and hints on how to proceed and what advice to give are included in the notes section.

Symptom sorter

This section attempts to list the possible signs and symptoms of common health concerns with which women present. This information has been obtained from a range of sources, and every attempt has been made to ensure that it is comprehensive and accurate. However, it is intended to serve only as a guide, and should not be a substitute for communication and liaison with colleagues. Furthermore, the signs and symptoms of a particular condition may vary from one individual to another. It is also recommended that the practitioner maintains current evidence-based knowledge through professional networks, journals and reputable Internet sites.

Menstrual symptoms

- **Absent periods**

- **Heavy periods**

- **Infrequent periods**

- **Inter-menstrual bleeding**

- **Irregular menstrual bleeding**

- **Painful periods**

Absent periods

Overview

The absence of periods is also known as amenorrhoea. Amenorrhoea can be classified as follows:

- primary – failure of menstruation to start
- secondary – periods stopping after a history of normal menstruation.

Specific areas for consideration when taking a history

- Contraception.
- Surgical history.
- Emotional upsets.
- Recent change in BMI and/or exercise regime.
- History of genetic abnormalities.
- Markers of androgenisation – hot flushes/sweats/hirsutism/raised BMI.

Differential diagnosis

Common	Occasional	Rare
• Pregnancy • Hormonal contraceptive injection and intrauterine system	• Weight loss/anorexia • Obesity • Excessive exercise • Stress • Post combined oral contraceptive • PCOS	• Chromosomal disorder (e.g Turner's syndrome) • Congenital cause (e.g. absence of uterus) • Ovarian failure • Pituitary disorders • Thyroid disorder • Tumour that is affecting hormone production

Possible investigations

- Urinary βHCG – to identify pregnancy.
- Blood tests for FSH/LH, prolactin and testosterone – to establish abnormal levels indicating ovarian failure or disturbance in pituitary function.
- TFTs – to identify a thyroid disorder.
- Karyotyping – if a chromosomal disorder is suspected.

To identify any structural abnormality or tumour:

- MRI
- pelvic USS
- laparoscopy
- hysteroscopy.

To ascertain the effect of abnormal hormone levels:

- bone density scan (if there is a history of more than 6 months of amenorrhoea).

Notes

- Bone mineral is laid down from early in life until we reach what is known as 'peak bone mass' (when the maximum amount of mineral is present in our bones) at around 30 years of age. The sex hormones, especially oestrogen, are important for the formation and maintenance of bone mineral content. Any factor that contributes to menstrual dysfunction can have a direct or indirect influence on bone mineral status due to the reduction in oestrogen levels.
- The Depo-Provera contraceptive injection can reduce the amount of circulating oestrogen in the body, which in turn decreases the amount of bone strength laid down in young women. Recent guidance from the Department of Health and the Faculty of Family Planning and Reproductive Health Care has advised that this method should only be used if no other contraceptive method is suitable, and that if it is used it should be reviewed with the client on a regular basis.[1]

Hazard warnings

- Always do a pregnancy test, even when the client's history would suggest that there is not a risk of pregnancy.
- Always calculate the BMI, as the client may be anorexic.
- Weight loss can cause amenorrhoea, so consider the causes of weight loss (e.g. thyrotoxicosis).

References

1 Clinical Effectiveness Unit. Contraceptive choices for young people. *J Fam Plan Reprod Health Care.* 2004; **30**: 237–51.

Heavy periods

Overview

Heavy periods, also known as menorrhagia, can be classified as follows:

- primary menorrhagia, in which the woman's periods have always been heavy
- secondary menorrhagia, in which the woman's periods were previously normal and have become heavy.

Clinically, menorrhagia is defined as total blood loss exceeding 80 ml per cycle, or a period that lasts for longer than 7 days.

Specific areas for consideration when taking a history

- Change in pattern and/or duration of periods.
- Medication (including contraceptives).
- Surgical history.
- Sexual health history.
- Family history of genetic abnormalities.

Differential diagnosis

Common	Occasional	Rare
• Fibroids	• IUD/Depo-Provera	• von Willebrand's disease
• STI	• PID	• Factor XI deficiency
• Anaemia	• Endometriosis	• Pituitary tumour
	• Endometrial polyps	• Endometrial cancer
	• Endometrial hyperplasia	
	• Hypothyroidism	
	• PCOS	

Possible investigations

- Bimanual examination – to detect the presence of abdominal masses, pelvic tenderness and adhesions.
- Speculum examination/proctoscopy – to facilitate sexual health screen.
- FBC – to detect anaemia.
- TFTs – to detect thyroid dysfunction.
- Pelvic USS – to identify any abdominal mass.
- Hysteroscopy/laparoscopy – to identify fibroids, polyps and endometrial deposits.
- Endometrial biopsy – when serious pathology is suspected.
- CT scan – to identify any pituitary abnormality.

Notes

Self-reporting regarding the heaviness of periods is subjective. Try to obtain an objective assessment by asking the patient to estimate the number of sanitary pads or tampons used.

Hazard warnings

- Establish whether there is irregular bleeding and/or post-coital bleeding as well as heavy bleeding, and refer the patient as appropriate.
- Significant bleeding can cause anaemia; always do a full blood count.
- Heavy bleeding with associated symptoms of pelvic tenderness and pain during intercourse can indicate endometriosis or chronic PID.

Infrequent periods

Overview

Infrequent menstruation, also known as oligomenorrhoea, is defined by a cycle length of between 6 weeks and 6 months in a woman who has previously had normal periods. At one extreme, it overlaps with normal, the cycles being ovulatory but infrequent, while at the other extreme there is amenorrhoea. Oligomenorrhoea can be caused by some of the disorders associated with amenorrhoea.

Specific areas for consideration when taking a history

- Medications, including contraceptives.
- Associated symptoms (e.g. menopausal symptoms, masculine features, breast discharge, impaired vision).
- Sexual health history.
- Gynaecological events or surgery.
- Recent changes in weight, diet or exercise regime.

Differential diagnosis

Common	Occasional	Rare

• PCOS
• Perimenopause
• POP
	• Pregnancy
	• Emotional/physical stress
	• Chronic illness
	• Poor nutrition
	• Eating disorders
	  (e.g. anorexia/obesity)
	• Diabetes
		• Oestrogen-secreting
		  tumours

Possible investigations

- Urinalysis – to detect possible diabetes.
- Urinary βHCG – to identify a pregnancy.
- FSH, LH, testosterone and oestradiol levels – to identify hormonal irregularities due to PCOS (high testosterone levels), oestrogen-secreting tumours (high oestrogen levels) and the menopause (high FSH and LH levels).
- Blood glucose levels – to detect diabetes.
- Pelvic USS – to identify polycystic ovaries.
- CT/MRI scan – to identify tumours.

Notes

- Periods are often light or widely spaced both in young women who have just started to menstruate and in women who are approaching the menopause. This is normal because in both instances the woman is not ovulating every month.
- Infrequent periods are common in young women, and only need to be investigated if the problem persists for more than 6 months.

Hazard warnings

- Always do a pregnancy test.
- Any post-menopausal vaginal bleeding is a cause for concern, and the patient should be referred to a gynaecologist immediately.
- Always calculate the BMI, as the patient may be anorexic.
- Weight loss can cause irregular periods, so consider the causes of weight loss (e.g. thyrotoxicosis).

Inter-menstrual bleeding

Overview

Inter-menstrual bleeding is also known as metrorrhagia. Any vaginal bleeding that is not normal menstrual bleeding or mid-cycle spotting may be abnormal and must be investigated. It may be a sign of a problem within the vagina, uterus or ovaries. This includes irregular or excessively heavy menstrual bleeding, and any vaginal bleeding in a woman who has passed the menopause.

Specific areas for consideration when taking a history

- Amount and occurrence of bleeding.
- Associated symptoms – fever, vaginal discharge and pain.
- Menstrual pattern.
- Obstetric history.
- Gynaecological history.
- Sexual health history.

Differential diagnosis

Common	Occasional	Rare
• STI • Pelvic infection • Cervical or uterine polyp • Uterine fibroid • Contraceptives – hormonal or IUD	• Vaginal/vulval injury • Ovarian cyst • Anovulatory cycles (PCOS) • Pregnancy • Miscarriage • Hypothyroidism • Cervical conisation/ cauterisation	• Uterine cancer • CIN

Possible investigations

- Urinary βHCG – to detect pregnancy.
- Blood tests:
  - FBC to detect possible anaemia with heavy bleeding
  - TFTs to detect possible thyroid dysfunction.
- Bimanual examination – to identify pelvic tenderness/adhesions.
- Speculum examination/proctoscopy – to examine the vagina and facilitate sexual health screen.
- Sexual health screen – to identify specific STIs.
- Cervical screening – to identify CIN.
- Pelvic USS – to identify any cysts/tumour.
- Colposcopy and hysteroscopy – a biopsy should be taken if significant pathology is suspected.

Notes

- The risk of malignancy increases with age.
- It is important to exclude bleeding from the rectum and blood in the urine.
- Keeping a menstrual diary could be useful for identifying the cause.

Hazard warnings

- Always do a pregnancy test.
- Always exclude sexually transmitted infection.
- Post-menopausal vaginal bleeding should prompt immediate referral to a gynaecologist.
- Consider direct referral for colposcopy.

Irregular menstrual bleeding

Overview

Irregular menstrual bleeding is far more likely to be due to a life event than to pathology. Taking a good history is vital.

Specific areas for consideration when taking a history

- Duration and pattern of symptoms.
- Associated symptoms (e.g. post-coital bleeding, menorrhagia).
- Medication (including contraceptives).
- Age.
- Life events.
- Sexual health history.

Differential diagnosis

Common	Occasional	Rare
• Perimenopause	• Weight gain	• Thyroid gland disorder
• Stress	• Weight loss	• Pituitary gland disorder
• Normal adolescence	• Vegetarian/vegan	• Hypothalamic amenorrhoea
• Travel	diet	
• Illness	• Anovulatory cycles	
• Excessive exercise	• Pregnancy	
• PCOS	• STI	
• Recently stopped COC		
• Breastfeeding		

Possible investigations

- Pregnancy test – to identify pregnancy.
- Bimanual examination – to detect signs of infection/pelvic masses.
- Speculum examination/proctoscopy – to facilitate a sexual health screen.
- Blood tests:
  - FBC to identify hormone levels
  - TFTs to identify abnormalities indicative of thyroid, pituitary or hypothalamic disorder.
- Sexual health screen – to identify specific STIs.

Notes

- In order to distinguish between inter-menstrual bleeding and irregular periods, it is best to ask the patient whether the bleeds feel like a period, with associated period-type symptoms.
- At both ends of a woman's menstrual life her periods may be irregular.

Hazard warnings

- Always do a pregnancy test.
- Calculate the BMI and ascertain whether there has been any weight change recently, as this may disrupt periods.
- Consider the influence of life events and travel on menstrual regularity.

Painful periods

Overview

If the discomfort of painful periods makes it virtually impossible to perform normal household, job- or school-related activities for a few days during each menstrual cycle, this is termed dysmenorrhoea, which can be classified as follows:

- primary dysmenorrhoea, in which periods have always been painful
- secondary dysmenorrhoea, in which pain is a new symptom.

Specific areas for consideration when taking a history

- Amount and duration of bleeding.
- Sexual health history.
- Cervical smear history.
- Contraception use.

Differential diagnosis

Common	Occasional	Rare
• Primary dysmenorrhoea – ovulatory cycles are established 6–12 months after menarche	• Uterine hypercontractility • Endometriosis • PID • IUD	• Endometrial polyps • Cervical pathology

Possible tests

- Pelvic examination – to identify polyps, tenderness, enlargement and fixity.
- Cervical smear/colposcopy – to identify cervical pathology.
- Speculum examination – to facilitate sexual health screen.

- Sexual health screen – to identify possible causes of PID.
- Pelvic USS – to detect uterine abnormalities.
- Hysteroscopy/laparoscopy – to identify adhesions/endometrial deposits.

Notes

- The following self-help measures can be useful.
  - Over-the-counter painkillers such as ibuprofen and paracetamol often help. There are also analgesic tablets available that contain the drug hyoscine (e.g. Feminax), which may help to prevent muscle contractions.
  - Moderate physical exercise can also be helpful for relieving pain, and may help to prevent period pain. Many women find that a hot-water bottle held against the abdomen or back is comforting. Self-heating patches or heat packs that can be warmed in a microwave are a convenient alternative.
- Younger patients may use the symptom of painful periods to obtain a prescription for the combined oral contraceptive pill.
- The pain may have no identifiable cause.

Hazard warnings

- If there are painful periods with associated symptoms such as heavy bleeding and abdominal pain/tenderness, consider the possibility of endometriosis or fibroids.
- Consider other possible causes, such as UTI and appendicitis.
- Pain thresholds can be affected by life events and the patient's psychological condition. Consider depression.

Hormonal changes

- **Early puberty**

- **Delayed puberty**

- **Hair loss**

- **Hirsutism**

- **Hot flushes**

- **Low libido**

- **Low mood**

- **Premenstrual symptoms**

- **Vaginal dryness**

Early puberty

Overview

Early puberty is also known as precocious puberty.

Definition

Early puberty is defined as breast and pubic hair development:

- before the age of 7 years in white individuals
- before the age of 6 years in black individuals

and as menarche before the age of 10 years.

   Referral is recommended if two of these signs are present in a child under 8 years of age.

Specific areas for consideration when taking a history

- Location and duration of symptoms.
- Menstrual history.

Differential diagnosis

Common	Occasional	Rare
• Benign unknown cause	• Head trauma • Tumour (of the brain or ovary) • Acquired (due to irradiation, surgery or infection, e.g. meningitis) • Hypothyroidism	• Inherited • Congenital (e.g. hydrocephalus, adrenal hyperplasia) • Russell–Silver syndrome and McCune–Albright syndrome

Possible investigations

- Physical examination – to identify visible signs of early puberty.
- Blood tests – FSH, LH, oestradiol, TSH, serum HCG – levels of which are raised in true precocious puberty.
- Screen for gonadotropin-secreting tumour.
- Left wrist radiograph to assess bone age.
- Consider MRI of the head to screen for pathology.
- MRI/CT scan for pituitary or other CNS lesion.
- Pelvic USS – to detect pathology.

Notes

- Visual field deficit suggests a pituitary mass.
- Increased body fat has been associated with early puberty in girls.

Hazard warnings

- Consider the possibility that the young person may not be the age that they say they are.
- Benign variants may be manifested as breast development in girls under 3 years of age, which spontaneously regresses, and pubic hair in both boys and girls under 7 years of age, due to adrenal androgen secretion in middle childhood (some authors consider that this may be a precursor to polycystic ovary syndrome, and recommend follow-up).

Delayed puberty

Overview

Delayed puberty is a term that is used to define the absence of pubertal changes in a girl aged 13 years or over or a boy aged 14 years or over, or the failure of developmental progression over a 2-year period. Delayed puberty occurs in about 2% of the adolescent population. Puberty may also be considered to be delayed in girls if the whole process is not complete in 4 years (or 4–5 years for boys), or if menarche has not occurred by the age of 16 years.

Specific areas for consideration in taking a history

- Medication.
- Chronic illness symptoms.
- Previous treatment or surgery.
- Eating patterns.
- Family medical history – height and age at onset of puberty.
- Signs of hormonal deficiency or excess.

Differential diagnosis

Common	Occasional	Rare
• Constitutional (natural) delay of puberty	• Hypothalamic suppression (e.g. systemic illness, anorexia nervosa)	• Chromosomal abnormalities (e.g. Klinefelter's syndrome, Turner's syndrome, Kallman's syndrome and Prader–Willi syndrome) • GnRH deficiency, pituitary lesion (e.g. craniopharyngioma) • Gonadal failure • Hypothyroidism • Hyperprolactinoma • Brain tumour

Possible investigations

- Examination of centiles in childhood – to identify normal late developers.
- Neurological examination – to identify Kallman's syndrome.
- Examination of body disproportion – to identify Kleinfelter's syndrome, Turner's syndrome and Prader–Willi syndrome.
- Blood levels – LH, FSH, oestradiol, testosterone, hydroxyprogesterone, TFTs and prolactin levels – to assess hormonal development.
- X-ray of hand – to assess bone age.
- CT or USS of pituitary, hypothalamus, adrenal glands and/or ovaries – to detect significant pathology.
- Chromosomal analysis – to identify possible syndrome.

Notes

- The timing of the beginning of puberty correlates better with a child's bone age than with their real chronological age, and puberty is unlikely to begin until a bone age of 11 years has been reached in girls, and 12 years in boys.

- Children with a constitutional delay in beginning puberty usually do not require treatment, and they will eventually start puberty and then progress through the stages of puberty normally. Some children, especially if they have hypogonadism, may benefit from treatment with sex hormones (testosterone for boys and oestrogen for girls), and should be referred to an endocrinologist/paediatrician.
- It is also important to evaluate and manage the psychological effects of beginning puberty late. Children in whom puberty is delayed are also usually shorter than other children of their own age, and together these factors can have a negative effect on the child.

Hazard warnings

- Consider the possibility that the young person may not be the age that they say they are.
- A good history can elicit whether the young person was delayed in other significant milestones, and whether there has been chronic illness or excessive exercise.
- Optic fundi, visual fields and sense of smell should be checked to look for evidence of a pituitary tumour.
- The commonest cause of delayed puberty in girls is Turner's syndrome (more than 80% of girls have a pathological cause of delayed puberty). Refer the patient for chromosomal analysis.

Hair loss

Overview

Hair loss, also known as alopecia, can be localised or diffuse, non-scarring (i.e. non-permanent) or scarring (permanent). Alopecia is an autoimmune disease that causes hair loss and can affect men, women and children of any age. The onset of hair loss is often sudden, random and frequently recurrent. Around 2% of the population will have alopecia to some degree during their lifetime. Men and women are equally affected. About 25% of people with alopecia have a family history of the disorder. Overall, 34–50% of people with alopecia areata recover within 1 year, almost every individual affected by the condition experiences more than one episode, and 14–25% progress to alopecia totalis or alopecia universalis.

Specific areas for consideration when taking a history

- Medication (including contraceptives).
- Associated symptoms (e.g. weight loss/gain, hot flushes, fever, tiredness).
- Obstetric factors (e.g. postpartum).
- Social factors (e.g. workplace, stressful events).

Differential diagnosis

Common	Occasional	Rare

• Pregnancy
• Contraception
• Menopause
• Emotional stress
• Physical stress
• Surgery
• Illness
• Anaemia
• Rapid weight change
• Fungal infection –
  Microsporum canis
  (mostly in children)
• Ringworm
• Traction alopecia (due
  to tight hairstyles)
• Diet – low iron, low
  protein
	• Androgenic alopecia
	  (female pattern baldness)
	• Psoriasis
	• Thyroid abnormalities
	• Alopecia areata
	  (autoimmune condition)
	• Trichotillomania
	  (compulsive pulling of hair)
	• Seborrhoeic dermatitis
	• Folliculitis
	• Mechanical trauma –
	  exposure to chemicals or
	  irradiation
	• Medications (high
	  doses of vitamin A,
	  antihypertensives, etc.)
	• Syphilis
		• Chronic discoid lupus
		  erythematosus
		• Lichen planus/
		  sclerosus
		• Scleroderma morphea
		• Neoplasms
		• Darier's disease
		• Aplasia cutis

Investigations

- MC&S – to detect scalp infection.
- Microscopic examination of scalp scrapings – to detect scalp infection.
- Blood tests:
  - TFTs to detect thyroid dysfunction
  - FBC to detect anaemia.
- Sexual health screen – to detect syphilis.
- Biopsy – to detect pathology.

Notes

- Alopecia can have a major psychological impact on the patient.

Hirsutism

Overview

Also known as hairiness, this condition is characterised by the growth of hairs over the cheeks, chin, beard area, moustache area, abdomen, breasts and back. It can be categorised as follows:

- hirsutism in which there is an underlying problem with the endocrine organs that results in increased hormone synthesis
- hirsutism in which there is no underlying problem.

Specific areas for consideration when taking a history

- Duration of symptom.
- Associated symptoms (e.g. menstrual pattern, weight).
- Medication.
- Age of onset.
- Rate of progression (sudden onset can indicate a tumour).
- Family history of hirsutism.

Differential diagnosis

Common	Occasional	Rare
• Idiopathic (genetic)	• PCOS • Medication	• Ovarian, adrenal or pituitary tumour (excessive production of male hormones) • Cushing's syndrome • Congenital adrenal hyperplasia

Possible tests

- Blood tests – serum testosterone, prolactin and cortisol to detect PCOS.
- Pelvic USS – to identify polycystic ovaries.

Notes

- Certain drugs (e.g. phenothiazines, androgen, minoxidil, diazoxide, steroids and phenytoin) can cause hirsutism.
- Hirsutism due to idiopathic causes or PCOS can be controlled by hormonal anti-androgens such as Dianette (which contains cyproterone acetate, which blocks testosterone activity).

Hazard warnings

- Sudden and severe onset of hairiness can indicate underlying pathology.
- Associated symptoms such as amenorrhoea and generally feeling unwell may indicate a hormone-secreting tumour.
- Associated headache and visual field disturbance suggest pituitary adenoma.

Hot flushes

Overview

Hot flushes are one of the most common symptoms of the climacteric or menopause, and are due to decreasing oestrogen levels. Therefore anything that interferes with oestrogen levels can cause hot flushes.

Specific areas for consideration when taking a history

- Other menopausal symptoms (e.g. dry vagina, night sweats, menstrual pattern).
- Medication.
- Surgical history.
- Lifestyle – stress, cigarettes, alcohol, exercise.

Differential diagnosis

Common	Occasional	Rare
• Menopause • Anxiety • Panic attacks	• Migraine • Alcohol/drugs • Association with food additives • Frey's syndrome • Side-effects of medication interfering with function of ovaries (e.g. chemotherapy)	• Early menopause – either natural or due to surgery • Carcinomas, tumours • Parkinson's disease

Possible investigations

- Blood tests – FSH, levels of which are high during the menopause.
- CT/X-ray – to detect pathology.

Notes

- Around 90% of hot flushes resolve within 2 years (associated with the menopause).
- It is useful to keep a diary to identify triggers.
- *Early menopause* refers to menopause (total cessation of periods for 12 months) before the age of 45 years. *Premature menopause* refers to menopause that occurs before the age of 40 years. If premature menopause occurs naturally – that is, not as a result of surgery, radiation treatment or chemotherapy – it is more commonly referred to as *premature ovarian failure*.

Hazard warnings

- Hot flushes associated with the following symptoms can indicate panic attacks: palpitations or a thumping heart, sweating and trembling, feeling short of breath, chest pains, feeling sick, feeling dizzy or faint, fear of dying.
- Brain tumours and spinal cord lesions can lead to vasomotor instability.
- In Frey's syndrome, re-nervation of the face leads to facial sweating when the salivary glands are stimulated. This should not be confused with the general effects of hot flushes.

Low libido

Overview

There are natural fluctuations in a woman's libido, which can be due to her normal menstrual rhythms, relationship difficulties, age or stress. Pathological causes of low libido are rare.

Specific areas for consideration when taking a history

- Details of symptom – is there a pattern or sudden onset?
- Other unusual symptoms (e.g. absent periods, anxiety).
- Medication (including contraceptives).
- Menstrual history.
- Obstetric history.
- Surgical history.
- Pregnancy risk.
- Drug use.
- Lifestyle.

Differential diagnosis

Common	Occasional	Rare
• Stress	• Cannabis use	• Low testosterone levels
• Pregnancy	• Medication	• Cushing's syndrome
• Postnatal depression	• Contraceptive method (anovulatory)	• Haemochromatosis
	• Surgery (e.g. hysterectomy)	• Pituitary cancer
	• Psychological factors (e.g. abuse)	

Possible investigations

- Urine βHCG – to detect pregnancy.
- Blood tests:
    - testosterone to detect low levels
    - pituitary hormones (prolactin, TSH and FSH) to detect pituitary dysfunction.
- CT/MRI scan – to detect any pituitary mass.
- Serum drug levels – to establish drug use.

Notes

- Keeping a diary of symptoms can be useful.

Hazard warnings

- Don't automatically look for a clinical cause. Explore the patient's lifestyle, stresses and emotional issues (e.g. fear of pregnancy, depression, postnatal depression, recent illness, homosexuality).
- Consider history of or current abuse that may cause fear of sex or low self-esteem.

Low mood

Overview

It is important to distinguish between low mood arising from normal life events and what may be clinical depression. Around 5–10% of people suffer from clinical depression in a given year, with 3–5% suffering from a milder form of depression. Women are at least twice as likely as men to experience episodes of severe clinical depression. Some studies have found that as many as 26% of women may have an episode of depression at some time in their lives, compared with approximately 12% of men.

Specific areas for consideration when taking a history

- Other associated symptoms (e.g. irritability, tiredness, weight changes).
- Obstetric history.
- Life events.
- Medication (including contraceptives).
- Drug use.

Differential diagnosis

Common	Occasional	Rare
• Contraceptive method (hormonal) • Grief/life events • Premenstrual syndrome • Menopause	• Drug abuse • Postviral syndrome • Hypothyroidism • Postnatal depression • Chronic fatigue syndrome • Diabetes • Fibromyalgia • Parkinson's disease • Side-effect of some medication	• Clinical depression • Side-effects of other conditions (e.g. Asperger's syndrome, autism, Addison's disease, Alzheimer's disease, lupus)

Possible investigations

- Blood tests:
  - TFTs to detect hypothyroidism
  - fasting glucose to determine how the body is processing sugar and detect diabetes.
- Urinalysis – to detect ketones indicative of diabetes.

Notes

- Diagnosis mainly depends on a good and thorough history.
- A mood diary could be useful for assessing the influence of the menstrual cycle.

Hazard warnings

- Do not underestimate low mood in the young adult. Because adolescence is stereotyped as a time of irritable moodiness, signs of teenage depression can be missed. Many instances of teenage depression lead to suicide attempts, and suicide is the third commonest cause of death among young adults aged between 15 and 25 years.
- Be aware that major depression has a high rate of coexistence with other disorders, including panic disorder, post-traumatic stress disorder, anxiety disorder, agoraphobia, social phobia and substance abuse.
- Ask about diet, as 'dieters' may experience low mood. This is linked to serotonin, the 'feel good' brain chemical that elevates mood, suppresses appetite and acts as a natural tranquilliser. A lack of dietary carbohydrates causes the brain to stop regulating serotonin levels. Serotonin is naturally produced after consumption of carbohydrates in the form of sweet and starchy foods. Although both men and women can experience low mood when cutting down on carbohydrates, women are more likely to feel the effects because they are known to have typically lower levels of serotonin in the brain than men.

Premenstrual symptoms

Overview

Premenstrual symptoms can be both physical and emotional. There is a spectrum of mild but identifiable symptoms. In *premenstrual dysphoric disorder* the symptoms are severe and disabling.

Specific areas for consideration when taking a history

- Medication history.
- Menstrual history.
- Smoking, diet and exercise.

Differential diagnosis

Common	Occasional	Rare
• Premenstrual syndrome/ tension • Stress (not a cause, but may make symptoms less manageable)	• Depression • Hypothyroidism • Anaemia • Premenstrual dysphoric disorder	• Clinical depression • Pituitary tumour

Possible investigations

- Blood tests:
  - TFTs to detect hypothyroidism
  - FBC to detect anaemia.
- Prospective symptom diary.
- CT scan – to detect pathology.

Notes

- Commonly these symptoms can be controlled by adopting a healthier way of life. In mild cases, advise the patient to take regular exercise, get enough sleep, eat healthy foods, stop smoking and find ways to manage stress. However, in more severe cases, drugs such as diuretics, ibuprofen, contraceptive pills or antidepressants may also be used.
- Another possibility is to suppress the menstrual cycle, and thus the hormonal fluctuations, by using medication that suppresses ovulation, such as the combined contraceptive pill, or contraceptive injection or implant.

Hazard warnings

Do not underestimate the impact of premenstrual syndrome on women's lives. The condition can increase the incidence of antisocial behaviour, accidents, illness and emotional crises in women, which in turn can affect their family, social and work relationships. Thus in addition to the physical discomfort and emotional disturbances associated with the condition itself, the patient may be overcome with guilt because of the effects of her premenstrual symptoms on those closest to her. This may contribute to the significant number of attempted suicides among premenstrual women.

Vaginal dryness

Overview

Vaginal dryness is a common condition that affects women of all ages. It is estimated that 10–40% of women who have reached the menopause have symptoms related to vaginal dryness. Other causes are usually related to factors that reduce oestrogen levels and thus decrease vaginal lubrication.

Specific areas for consideration when taking a history

- Medication (including contraceptives).
- Age.
- Associated symptoms (e.g. hot flushes, irregular or absent periods).
- Obstetric history.
- Sexual health history.

Differential diagnosis

Common	Occasional	Rare
• Normal ageing	• Diabetes – neuropathy	• Prolactinoma
• Menopause	• Chemical allergy	• Decreased ovarian
• Postpartum	• Trichomoniasis infection	function due to
• Breastfeeding	• Vaginal trauma	chemotherapy and/or
• Yeast infection	• Vaginal douching	radiotherapy
• Bacterial infection	• Surgery (e.g. hysterectomy)	• Sjögren's syndrome
	• Cigarette smoking	

Possible investigations

- Vaginal speculum examination – to detect dermal causes.
- Speculum examination – to facilitate sexual health screen.
- Sexual health screen – to identify specific STIs.
- Blood tests:
  – blood sugar levels to detect diabetes
  – prolactin levels to detect prolactinoma.
- Urinalysis – to detect ketones indicative of diabetes.

Notes

Several natural remedies are available, and some researchers believe that adding certain items to the diet may help to increase moisture levels in the vagina. However, more research is needed to determine the safety and effectiveness of these approaches. Examples of natural remedies include the following:

- isoflavones (plant oestrogens) – these compounds are found in soybeans and soy products, and may produce a weak oestrogen-like effect
- black cohosh (also called snakeroot or bugbane) – this plant may help to reduce some menopausal symptoms, including vaginal dryness. It should not be used if the patient is pregnant, nursing, or taking a medication that can harm the liver.

Hazard warnings

- Don't forget to ask the patient whether they use products on the genital area (e.g. perfume, douches, soap) which may cause a local allergic reaction and contribute to a lack of vaginal moisture.
- Don't be afraid to carry out a genital examination. It may highlight skin conditions such as psoriasis, or the presence of fungal or bacterial infection.

Sexual health

- **Acute pelvic pain**

- **Anogenital lesions**

- **Anogenital lumps and bumps**

- **Bleeding after sex**

- **Chronic pelvic pain**

- **Genital pain**

- **Painful intercourse (dyspareunia)**

- **Vaginal discharge**

- **Vaginal itch**

- **Vulval swelling**

Acute pelvic pain

Overview

Many women experience pain in their pelvic region at some stage in their life. However, finding the cause of pelvic pain can be a long process. Often there is more than one reason for the pain, and its exact source can be difficult to detect. Acute pelvic pain often has a single cause. This type of pain may be a warning that something is wrong, such as an infection, ovarian cysts or an ectopic pregnancy.

Specific areas for consideration when taking a history

- Duration and location of pain.
- Associated symptoms (e.g. fever, vaginal discharge).
- Medication (including contraceptives).
- Menstrual history.
- Sexual health history.

Differential diagnosis

Common	Occasional	Rare
• PID	• Pelvic abscess	• Perforation following IUD insertion
• UTI	• Endometriosis	• Carcinoma
• Miscarriage	• Pelvic congestion	• Fibroid degeneration
• Ectopic pregnancy		• Hernia
• Ovarian cysts		

Possible investigations

- Urinary βHCG – to detect pregnancy.
- Blood βHCG – to detect pregnancy.
- Urinalysis/MSU – to detect UTI.
- Speculum examination/proctoscopy – to facilitate sexual health screen.
- Bimanual examination – to identify pelvic tenderness and adhesions.
- STI screen – to identify any STI.
- Pelvic USS – to detect ovarian cysts or possible ectopic pregnancy.
- Laparoscopy – to identify endometriosis.
- Biopsy – to eliminate pathology.

Notes

- Consider psychosexual issues.
- Consider constipation and irritable bowel syndrome.

Hazard warnings

- Severe unilateral pain and tenderness around 6 weeks after the last menstrual period suggest ectopic pregnancy, even with no bleeding. The patient should be admitted urgently.

Anogenital lesions

Overview

Because genital lesions or sores often have an adverse effect on a person's self-image, many individuals do not seek prompt medical care. A range of conditions can produce lesions. Approximately 10% of lesions become superinfected with bacteria or *Candida*.

Specific areas for consideration when taking a history

- Location and duration of lesions.
- Medication (including contraceptives).
- Sexual health history.

Differential diagnosis

Common	Occasional	Rare
• Human papilloma virus	• Furuncle	• Granuloma inguinale
• Herpes simplex virus	• Hydradenitis supparativa	• Lymphogranuloma
• Molluscum	• Scabies	venereum
• Ulcer	• Syphilis	• Behçet's disease
• Boil	• Chancroid	• Skin cancer
	• Chickenpox	• HIV/AIDS
	• Erythema multiforme	

Possible investigations

- Speculum examination/proctoscopy – to facilitate sexual health screen.
- Sexual health screen – to identify specific STIs.
- Swabs – MC&S and viral, to detect any superinfection or HSV.
- Biopsy – to eliminate pathology.

Notes

- Lesions can make it painful to urinate or defecate. Warm water poured over the urethra while urinating can ease the pain. Painkillers and topical anaesthesia may also help.
- A pregnant woman with primary HSV can transmit the virus to her baby, and this carries a significant morbidity and mortality risk. In such cases a Caesarean section may be the preferred route of delivery.

Hazard warnings

- Take a history of travel and sexual contact while abroad, as there could be a number of tropical causes.
- A client with a single persistent vulval lesion should be referred to a genito-urinary specialist, as significant disease is likely.
- Consider the possibility of undiagnosed diabetes in severe cases of *Candida*.
- Consider the possibility of abuse if anogenital lesions are present in a minor.

Anogenital lumps and bumps

Overview

There are many causes of genital lumps and bumps. It is important not to confuse normal anatomical variants with genital warts. In many women, the entrance to the vagina normally feels lumpy. This lumpiness is the remains of the hymen (which stretches across the entrance in young girls). A woman who has given birth to a child, and who needed stitches afterwards, may also be left with a lumpy scar at the vaginal opening.

Specific areas for consideration in taking a history

- Nature and duration of symptom.
- Medication (including contraceptives).
- Sexual health history.
- Obstetric history.

Differential diagnosis

Common	Occasional	Rare
• Human papilloma virus • Folliculitis	• Molluscum • Abscess • Skin tag • Lice • Scabies • Dermatoses • Haemorrhoids	• Tumours

Possible investigations

- Bimanual examination/speculum examination/proctoscopy – to facilitate sexual health screen.
- Sexual health screen – to identify specific STIs.
- Colposcopy/biopsy – to identify cervical pathology and genital pathology.

Notes

- If vulval intra-epithelial neoplasia (VIN) is diagnosed, there is a greater than 10% risk of neoplasia elsewhere, generally cervical. Therefore if VIN is diagnosed, an examination of the cervix and breasts should be undertaken.
- There is a particularly noticeable increase in genital warts among teenagers. In women, about 60% of genital warts are in the 16–24 years age group.

Hazard warnings

- Take a history of travel and sexual contact while abroad, as there could be a number of tropical causes.
- Consider the possibility of abuse if STI are present in a minor.

Bleeding after sex

Overview

Post-coital bleeding (PCB) is non-menstrual bleeding that occurs immediately after sexual intercourse. It can be due to a benign cause such as cervical ectropion. However, it is often caused by an infection. Infections can cause the cervix to become inflamed and more prone to bleeding. A diagnosis is usually reached by a process of elimination.

Specific areas for consideration when taking a history

- Duration of symptom.
- Medication (including contraceptives).
- Previous surgical interventions.
- Gynaecological history.
- Cervical cytology history.
- Obstetric history.
- Sexual health history.

Differential diagnosis

Common	Occasional	Rare
• Cervical ectropion • Ovulation (mid-cycle bleeding)/ mittelschmerz • Cervicitis	• Cervical lesion • Polyp • PID • Atrophic vaginitis (post-menopausal) • Hypothyroidism • Hyperthyroidism	• Malignancy • Endometriosis

Possible investigations

- Bimanual/speculum examination and proctoscopy – to visualise a polyp, facilitate a sexual health screen and identify uterine and tubal tenderness.
- Sexual health screen – to identify specific STIs.
- Cervical smear – to detect pathology.
- Blood tests – TFTs to detect thyroid dysfunction.
- Colposcopy/hysteroscopy and biopsy – to detect pathology.

Notes

- If in doubt, establish that the bleeding is from the vagina, not from the rectum or in the urine. Insertion of a tampon will confirm whether blood is present in the vagina.

Hazard warnings

- Older women who complain of PCB should have a colposcopy irrespective of the smear result. Any post-menopausal bleeding should be assumed to be due to endometrial carcinoma until proved otherwise.

Chronic pelvic pain

Overview

Pelvic pain is one of the commonest reasons for referral to a gynaecology clinic, and for a woman consulting her GP in the first place. It is defined as chronic if it has been present for three or more cycles. The difference between chronic pelvic pain and expected period pain is one of intensity and duration.

Specific areas for consideration when taking a history

* Duration, location and nature of pain.
* Medication (including contraceptives).
* Menstrual history.
* Obstetric history.
* Sexual health history.

Differential diagnosis

Common	Occasional	Rare
• Endometriosis • Chronic PID • Irritable bowel syndrome • Physiological ovulation pain (mittelschmerz, dysmenorrhoea)	• Recurrent UTI • Mechanical low back pain • Uterovaginal prolapse • Benign tumours (ovarian cyst, fibroids)	• Malignant tumours (ovary, cervix, bowel) • Diverticulitis • Lower colonic cancer • Inflammatory bowel disease • Subacute bowel obstruction • Pelvic congestion

Possible investigations

* MSU – to detect UTI.
* Bimanual examination – to detect pelvic tenderness and adhesions.
* Speculum examination/proctoscopy – to facilitate sexual health screen.
* Sexual health screen – to identify specific STIs.
* Pelvic ultrasound scan – to detect cysts and possible ectopic pregnancy.
* Laparoscopy – to identify endometriosis and pathology.
* Biopsy – to eliminate pathology.
* CT/MRI scan – to identify bowel obstruction.

Notes

* Consider psychological causes of chronic pelvic pain.
* A forgotten IUD can cause cyclical pelvic pain.
* If the pain is associated with periods and is secondary dysmenorrhoea, it is more likely to have a pathological cause.

Hazard warnings

- Ovarian cancer almost always presents late. Always perform a pelvic examination in women with chronic pelvic pain.
- Someone who has been the victim of sexual abuse is more likely to experience chronic pelvic pain.

Genital pain

Overview

Genital pain can be a symptom of many conditions. A very careful and detailed history should be taken to establish the exact nature and location of the pain. This information will then inform the decision as to which investigations are required.

Specific areas for consideration when taking a history

- Duration and location of symptom (internal/external).
- Is the pain worse with sexual intercourse?
- Medication (including contraceptives).
- Menstrual history.
- Previous surgical interventions.
- Gynaecological history.
- Cervical cytology history.
- Obstetric history.
- Sexual health history.

Differential diagnosis

Common	Occasional	Rare
• Vaginal infection/STI	• Vulval abscess	• Fissure/sinus
• Ulceration	• Vaginismus	• Tumours
• Menstrual pain	• Vulvodynia	
• Referred bowel pain	• Trauma	
• UTI	• Ectopic pregnancy	
	• Fibroids/cysts	
	• Ovulation pain	
	• Haemorrhoids	

Possible investigations

- Urinary βHCG/serum βHCG – to detect pregnancy.
- MSU – to detect UTI.
- Bimanual examination – to detect pelvic tenderness and adhesions.
- Speculum examination/proctoscopy – to facilitate sexual health screen.

- Sexual health screen – to identify specific STIs.
- Cervical cytology – to identify CIN.
- Pelvic USS to – detect cysts and possible ectopic pregnancy.
- Laparoscopy – to identify pathology.
- Biopsy – to eliminate pathology.

Notes

- Consider psychological causes of genital pain.

Painful intercourse (dyspareunia)

Overview

Dyspareunia may be categorised as follows:

- superficial – pain confined to the introitus (vaginal entrance)
- deep – pain experienced deep in the pelvis during intercourse
- orgasmic – pain during orgasm
- post-coital – pain following coitus.

Specific areas for consideration when taking a history

- Duration and nature of pain (e.g. external/deep).
- Medication (including contraceptives).
- Sexual health history.
- Obstetric history.
- Menstrual history.
- Life events.
- Attitude towards sexual intercourse.

Differential diagnosis

Common	Occasional	Rare
• Poor sexual stimulation • Vaginismus • Vulvovaginitis (bacterial vaginosis, thrush, *Trichomonas vaginalis*, ulceration, bartholinitis) • Vaginal dryness (psychological, menopausal) • Endometriosis (cyclical pain) • PID/cervicitis	• Perineal repair postpartum • Cystitis • Urethritis • Pelvic adhesions (post surgical, PID) • Fibroid • Vaginal atrophy (post-menopausal or due to infrequent sexual intercourse) • Anal fissure • Adenomyosis	• Ovarian cyst/ tumour • Unruptured hymen • Perineal abscess • Vulval dysplasia • Prolapsed ovaries • Allergy to sperm

Possible investigations

- Urinalysis/MSU – to detect urethritis.
- Bimanual examination – to detect pelvic tenderness and adhesions.
- Speculum examination/proctosopy – to facilitate sexual health screen.
- Sexual health screen – to identify specific STIs.
- Pelvic USS – to detect cysts and possible ectopic pregnancy.
- Laparoscopy – to identify pathology.
- Biopsy – to eliminate pathology.

Notes

- Consider psychological causes of painful intercourse. These include fear, ignorance, vaginismus, previous painful intercourse and relationship problems.
- Dyspareunia with sudden onset is likely to have an organic cause. Chronic dyspareunia is more likely to have a psychosexual cause.
- Consider the possibility of inadequate lubrication due to either lack of arousal or sexual phobia.
- Superficial dyspareunia is usually caused by infection, vaginismus or atrophy. Deep dyspareunia may be caused by pelvic pathology.
- The patient who complains that her vagina feels too small to accommodate her partner's penis probably has vaginismus.

Hazard warnings

- Cyclical dyspareunia with generalised pelvic pain and heavy painful periods suggests endometriosis or PID, and the patient should be referred for a gynaecological opinion.
- Pelvic tumours are rare, but consider this possibility in older women with sudden-onset dyspareunia.
- Consider vulval dysplasia, rather than atrophic vaginitis, in menopausal or perimenopausal women who complain of persistent superficial dyspareunia

Vaginal discharge

Overview

Vaginal discharge is usually a symptom of the reproductive years, and is influenced by the menstrual cycle, use of the oral contraceptive pill, pregnancy and sexual activity.

Specific areas for consideration when taking a history

- Duration, colour, consistency and smell of discharge.
- Medication (including contraceptives).
- Sexual health history.
- Cervical screening history.
- Obstetric history.

Differential diagnosis

Common	Occasional	Rare
• Excessive normal discharge • Thrush • Bacterial vaginosis • *Trichomonas vaginalis* • Cervicitis due to gonorrhoea, chlamydia or herpes	• Cervical ectropion • Cervical polyp • Foreign body • IUD • Bartholinitis	• Neoplasia • Fibroid (sloughing) • Pyometra • Pelvic fistula

Possible investigations

- Speculum examination – to facilitate a sexual health screen.
- STI screen – to identify any causative organisms.
- Cervical screen, colposcopy and biopsy – to detect pathology.

Notes

- Vaginal discharge is uncommon before puberty. Consider discreet assessment for non-accidental injury/abuse.
- In post-menopausal women a vaginal discharge should always be investigated, as malignancy is one of the most likely causes.

Hazard warnings

- Always eliminate *Chlamydia trachomatis* in women who have had unprotected sexual intercourse. Refer the patient for a GUM screen.
- Vaginal discharge is uncommon in a minor. Consider the possibility of abuse or the presence of a foreign body.
- Vaginal discharge in post-menopausal women is unusual, and malignancy is one of the likeliest causes.

Vaginal itch

Overview

Usually associated with vaginal soreness, this is a very common symptom in women.

Specific areas for consideration when taking a history

- Medication (including contraceptives).
- Menstrual history.
- Obstetric history.
- Sexual health history.
- Hygiene.

Differential diagnosis

Common	Occasional	Rare
• *Candida* (thrush) • *Trichomonas vaginalis* • Soaps, bubble baths, etc. • Trauma (i.e. reduced lubrication during sexual intercourse) • Atrophic vaginitis (usually soreness)	• Diabetes (associated with recurrent thrush) • Irritation due to incontinence • Psoriasis • Lichen planus • Infestations	• Lichen sclerosus • Leukoplakia • Carcinoma • Jaundice • Psychosexual cause

Possible investigations

- Urinalysis – to detect diabetes.
- Blood tests:
  - LFT to assess liver function
  - fasting blood sugar to detect diabetes.
- Sexual health screen – to identify *Candida* or *Trichomonas vaginalis* or to visualise dermatological causes or mites.
- Biopsy – to detect any pathology.

Notes

- Bear in mind that scratching and self-medication can distort the appearance of the vulva/vagina.
- Occasionally vulval itching can be a manifestation of a general skin disorder such as eczema or psoriasis.
- Recurrent thrush can be a particular cause for concern for women. It is important to spend time assessing the particular case, exploring the woman's perception of the problem, possible therapeutic interventions and other self-help factors.

Hazard warnings

- Dysplasias and some carcinomas can cause intense irritation. Always examine the patient, and refer for biopsy as appropriate.
- Consider diabetes in cases of recurrent infection with *Candida*.
- Consider STIs such as herpes and warts. Examine the patient and refer for a general GUM screen as appropriate.

Vulval swelling

Overview

Vaginal infections often affect not only the vagina but also the vaginal opening and the skin around it, causing itching, swelling and pain.

Specific areas for consideration when taking a history

- Menstrual history.
- Sexual health history.
- Hygiene.

Differential diagnosis

Common	Occasional	Rare
• Thrush	• Eczema	• Vaginal cancer
• *Trichomonas vaginalis*	• Hives	• Reiter's syndrome
• Bacterial vaginosis	• Atrophic vaginitis	• Vulval TB
• Herpes simplex virus	(menopause)	• Condylomata
• Human papilloma virus	• Foreign body in vagina	accuminata
• Vulval skin allergy	• Gonorrhoea	• Vulval intra-epithelial
(dermatitis)	• PID	neoplasia
• Vulval skin injury	• Bartholin's cyst	• Vulval leukoplakia
• Pubic lice		(lichen sclerosus)

Possible investigations

- Vaginal examination – to visualise any injury or skin infection.
- Bimanual examination – to detect pelvic tenderness in PID.
- Speculum examination – to visualise any foreign body and facilitate a sexual health screen.
- Sexual health screen – to identify specific STIs.
- Biopsy – to identify any pathology.

Notes

- As with vaginal itching, scratching and self-medication can distort the appearance of the vulva/vagina.
- If a lump is not obvious on examination, examine the patient while standing, as this may reveal a hernia, varicocele or prolapse.

Hazard warnings

- A persistent lump in the vulva should always be referred for biopsy to exclude carcinoma.
- A woman with genital warts may have a coexisting STI, and should be referred for a GUM screen.

Breast symptoms

- **Breast lump**

- **Breast pain**

- **Nipple discharge**

Breast lump

Overview

The vast majority of breast lumps are benign. All women have lumpy breasts, and many of the lumps that women find are areas of normal breast tissue which can become more prominent and lumpy just before a period.

Specific areas for consideration when taking a history

- Consistency, tenderness and duration of lump.
- Associated symptoms (e.g. discharge, fever).
- Age – carcinoma is more likely after the menopause.
- Predisposing events (e.g. trauma).
- Timing (e.g. cyclical).
- Medication (including contraceptives).
- Obstetric history.
- Surgical history.

Differential diagnosis

Common	Occasional	Rare
• Breastfeeding – mastitis abscess, infections in sebaceous glands	• Non-infective mastitis • Fibroadenoma (discreet lump) • Lipoma • Lax cyst • Fibroadenosis – may produce painful lumpy breast • Fibroadenotic cyst (painless)	• Carcinoma (painless, poorly defined margin, evidence of tethering) • Galactocele • Other cysts • Trauma (fat necrosis) (painless)

Possible investigations

- Examination – to assess the lump.
- USS – to locate any pathology.
- Mammogram – to locate any pathology.
- Aspiration – to obtain a sample for analysis.
- Biopsy – to identify any pathology.

Notes

- Women who have breast cysts are at slightly increased risk of developing breast cancer, but this risk is not considered to be significant.
- If on examination it is difficult to identify a lump, refer the woman rather than delaying, as she will be anxious.
- A mass appearing after trauma may be due to fat necrosis. Check it again after a few weeks and refer the patient if it has not resolved.

Hazard warnings

- Associated signs such as skin dimpling, local flattening and nipple changes indicate cancer until proved otherwise.
- In post-menopausal women a breast lump will almost certainly be cancerous, and an urgent referral is required.

Breast pain

Overview

Breast pain is a common symptom in up to two-thirds of women, and is usually associated with cyclical hormonal changes.

Specific areas for consideration when taking a history

- Duration, type and location of pain.
- Other symptoms (e.g. fever).
- Medication (including contraceptives).
- Surgical history.

Differential diagnosis

Common	Occasional	Rare
• Cyclical mastalgia – part of normal changes in menstrual cycle • Pregnancy • Onset of puberty or menopause • Oestrogen therapy • Breastfeeding – cracked nipple infection, nipple thrush	• Periareolar infection (duct infection) • Peripheral infection (associated with pre-existing conditions, e.g. diabetes, trauma) • Breast abscess • Skin-associated breast infection (e.g. due to obesity, poor hygiene, radiotherapy, surgery) • Fibroadenoma • Cyst • Shingles	• Tender costochondral junctions (Tietze's syndrome) • Fibroadenosis • Carcinoma (rarely painful) • Mondor's disease (following trauma) • Cervical/thoracic spondylosis • Bornholm disease • Lung disease • Gallstones • Thoracic outlet syndrome • Granulomatous lobular mastitis • Rare breast infections (e.g. TB, syphilis, actinomycosis, helminthis infection, viral infection)

Possible investigations

- Examination – to locate superficial infection.
- Urinalysis – βHCG to detect pregnancy.
- MC&S – to identify infection.
- USS, X-ray, mammography and biopsy – to identify pathology.
- Heaf test – to detect tuberculosis antibodies.

Notes

- A pain chart that is filled in for a couple of months can be useful.
- If the pain is related to exertion in an older woman, angina could be a possibility.

Hazard warnings

- Consider pregnancy as a cause.
- A breastfeeding woman with unilateral breast pain and flu-type symptoms may be developing mastitis. Treat early to avoid the development of an abscess.

Nipple discharge

Overview

Nipple discharge is the third commonest breast complaint for which women seek medical attention, after lumps and breast pain. A woman's breasts show some degree of fluid secretion activity throughout most of adulthood. The difference between lactating (milk-producing) and non-lactating breasts lies mainly in the amount of secretion and, to a lesser degree, in the chemical composition of the fluid. In non-lactating women, small plugs of tissue block the nipple ducts and prevent the nipple from discharging fluid. During breast self-examination, fluid may be expressed from the breasts.

Specific areas for consideration when taking a history

- Colour and amount of discharge, whether both breasts are affected, whether there is one opening or multiple ones, whether discharge is spontaneous or only occurs in response to mechanical stimulation.
- Other symptoms (e.g. hot flushes, dry vagina, etc.).
- Medication (including contraceptives).
- Recent chest injury.

Differential diagnosis

Common	Occasional	Rare
• Pregnancy (milky) • Mechanical stimulation of breasts (after breastfeeding) • Stress causing hyperprolactinaemia • Breast infection (in lactating women)	• Hyperprolactinaemia leading to galactorrhoea (milky) • Perimenopausal (brown/green) • Mammary duct ectasia (brown/green) • Underactive thyroid (hypothyroidism) • Antidepressants • Combined oral contraceptive • Tranquillisers • Fibroadenosis (brown/green) Fibrocystic changes	• Carcinoma (bloodstained) • Intraductal papilloma (bloodstained) • Prolactinoma/ cerebral tumour • Ectopic prolactin synthesis • Paget's disease of the breast

Possible investigations

- Urinary βHCG – to detect pregnancy.
- Breast examination – to assess whether there is any infection.
- MC&S – to identify specific infection.
- Prolactin levels – to detect abnormal levels.
- USS – to detect any pathology.

- Mammogram – to detect any pathology.
- CT scan – to detect cerebral mass.
- Assess visual field – to check for possible pituitary tumour.
- Biopsy – to identify pathology.

Notes

- If discharge is bilateral, serious breast disease is unlikely.
- Consider pregnancy with bilateral discharge.

Hazard warnings

- If a premenopausal woman is amenorrhoeic with bilateral discharge, and pregnancy has been excluded, consider hyperprolactinaemia.
- Women over 40 years of age with new breast discharge should be referred in order to exclude serious pathology.
- Bright red blood discharging from one orifice suggests duct papilloma or carcinoma.

Urinary symptoms

- **Blood in the urine**

- **Excessive urination**

- **Frequency of urination**

- **Pain on urination**

- **Urinary incontinence**

Blood in the urine

Overview

Blood in the urine is also known as haematuria. A trace amount of blood in the urine is normal. The average person with a healthy urinary tract excretes about 1 million red blood cells (RBC) in the urine each day. This amount of blood is not visible, and is not considered to be haematuria. An abnormal amount of blood in the urine can be either acute (new, occurring suddenly) or chronic (ongoing, long-term). Blood in the urine can be caused by any condition that results in infection, inflammation or injury of the urinary system.

Specific areas for consideration when taking a history

- Associated symptoms.
- Trauma.
- Lifestyle/travel.
- Sexual health history.

Differential diagnosis

Common	Occasional	Rare
• UTI	• Injury	• Kidney stones, cysts or disease
• Cystitis	• Vaginal bleeding	• Bladder cancer
• Strenuous exercise	• Kidney infection	• TB
• STI	• Nephritis	• Bilharzia
	• Pyelonephritis	
	• Bladder polyp	

Possible investigations

- Urinalysis – to detect signs of urine infection.
- MSU – to identify specific infection.
- U&Es – to identify imbalance due to kidney malfunction.
- Heaf test – to assess tuberculosis antibodies.
- CT scan – to identify pathology.
- Cystoscopy – to visualise pathology.
- Renal biopsy – to identify pathology.

Notes

- Typically, microscopic haematuria indicates damage to the upper urinary tract (kidneys), whereas visible blood indicates damage to the lower urinary tract (ureters, bladder or urethra). However, this is not always the case.
- Sometimes no cause can be found for blood in the urine.

Hazard warnings

- Painless frank haematuria is an ominous sign and can indicate malignancy.
- Recent onset of recurrent cystitis with haematuria in the elderly may be caused by a bladder tumour.

Excessive urination

Overview

Excessive urination is also known as polyuria, and is usually associated with excessive thirst (polydipsia). It is defined as the release of abnormally large amounts of urine (for an adult, at least 2.5 litres per day).

Specific areas for consideration when taking a history

- Associated symptoms (thirst, abdominal pain, vomiting).

Differential diagnosis

Common	Occasional	Rare
• UTI	• Diabetes	• Compulsive water
• Chronic renal failure	• Potassium depletion	drinking
• Hyperparathyroidism	(e.g. due to diarrhoea	• Fanconi's syndrome
• Hypokalaemia secondary	and/or vomiting)	
to certain medication	• Cushing's syndrome	
(e.g. diuretics)	• Sickle-cell anaemia	
• Hypercalcaemia		

Possible tests

- Blood tests:
  - FBC and U&Es to identify any imbalance in renal function
  - serum calcium levels to identify hypocalcaemia
  - sickle to diagnose sickle-cell anaemia
  - fasting glucose levels to identify diabetes.
- Urinalysis – to identify signs of UTI and diabetes.
- MSU – to identify specific infection.
- Renal USS – to identify pathology.
- Cystoscopy – to visualise pathology.
- Biopsy – to identify pathology.

Notes

- It is important to distinguish between excessive urination and urinary frequency, as the causes are very different.

Hazard warnings

- If urinalysis is negative for sugar, consider diabetes insipidus or hypercalcaemia.
- Weight loss and cough in a smoker with polyuria suggest a possible ACTH-secreting tumour. Refer the patient for a chest X-ray.
- If urinalysis reveals glucose and ketones in a known diabetic, arrange for an urgent assessment and possible admission for stabilisation.
- Renal disease is likely in patients with polydipsia who have blood and protein on urinalysis.

Frequency of urination

Overview

Increased urinary frequency is defined as the need to urinate more often than usual. Increased urgency is a sudden, compelling urge to urinate, along with discomfort in the bladder. More commonly known as *cystitis*, urinary frequency can be caused by inflammation of the lining of the bladder. Infection may be caused by bacteria, viruses or fungi.

Specific areas for consideration when taking a history

- Duration of symptoms.
- Other urinary symptoms – burning sensation (inside indicates cystitis, outside indicates urethritis or vaginitis), blood in urine and fever.
- Last menstrual period, possible pregnancy or actual pregnancy.
- Contraceptive method.
- Sexual health history.
- History of UTIs.

Differential diagnosis

Common	Occasional	Rare
• Acute cystitis	• Acute urethritis	• Herpes simplex virus
• Diuretics (e.g. drinks containing caffeine)	• Acute vaginitis	• Urinary tract abnormality
• Sexual intercourse (mechanical introduction of pathogens into bladder)	• Pregnancy (effect of progestogen on smooth muscle allows relaxation of urethral meatus)	• Bladder/urethral stones
	• Diabetes (urinary glucose impairs leucocyte phagocytosis)	• Pelvic space-occupying lesion (e.g. fibroid, ovarian cyst, carcinoma)
	• Diaphragm use (pH change, mechanical obstruction)	• Bladder tumour
	• Detrusor muscle instability (activation of voiding reflex before bladder is completely filled)	• Post-radiotherapy fibrosis
	• Renal TB	

Possible investigations

- Urinalysis – for signs of UTI, pregnancy or diabetes.
- MSU culture – to identify specific infection.
- Speculum examination – to facilitate sexual health screen.
- Sexual health screen – to identify specific STIs.
- Blood test fasting glucose levels – to identify diabetes.
- USS – to identify pathology.
- Intravenous pyelography – to identify urinary system pathology.
- Cystoscopy – to visualise pathology.
- Urodynamic investigations – to identify urinary system pathology.

Notes

- Together, urinary frequency and urgency are classic signs of UTI. Since inflammation reduces the bladder's capacity to hold urine, even small amounts of urine cause discomfort.
- Anxiety can cause urinary frequency. It is typically long-term and increases with stress. There is nil on urinalysis.

Hazard warnings

- Appendicitis can cause mild frequency and pyuria.
- Consider pregnancy.
- Recent onset of recurrent cystitis with haematuria in the elderly may be caused by a bladder tumour.

Pain on urination

Overview

Pain on urination is called dysuria. This painful, burning sensation is a common complaint in young women. It usually indicates UTI, but can also indicate an STI.

Specific areas for consideration when taking a history

- Duration and description of pain (inside indicates trigonitis, outside indicates vaginitis).
- Associated symptoms – frequency, burning sensation, blood.
- Medication (including contraceptives).
- Sexual health history.

Differential diagnosis

Common	Occasional	Rare

• Cystitis
• Vaginitis – thrush/
  Trichomonas vaginalis
• Urethritis – chlamydia,
  gonorrhoea, herpes
  simplex virus
• UTI
• STI
• Diaphragm use
	• Trauma
	• Stone in urinary tract or
	  bladder
	• Irritation secondary to
	  radiotherapy
	• Obstructive uropathy
		• Urinary TB
		• Underlying aetiology –
		  tumours

Investigations

- Urinalysis – to identify the presence of a UTI.
- MSU culture – to identify the specific infection and appropriate antibiotics.
- STI screen – to identify sexually transmitted pathogens.
- USS – to visualise stones or a structural defect.
- Cystoscopy – to visualise pathology or a structural defect.
- IV pyelography – to visualise a structural defect.

Notes

- Dysuria with frequency and urgency suggests cystitis. Women usually experience internal discomfort (located in the urethra and bladder), rather than external discomfort such as the labial irritation associated with vaginitis.
- Dysuria associated with symptoms of PID, occurring around 1 to 2 weeks after intercourse or noted just at the start of urination, suggests urethritis.
- Associated fever, myalgia and headache suggest acute pyelonephritis or primary genital herpes as the cause of dysuria.
- Consider examining the client, as vulval infections can cause pain during urination.

Hazard warnings

- STIs can cause dysuria. Refer the patient for a GUM screen.
- Consider pelvic pathology, such as ovarian cysts which may press on the ureter and cause dysuria.
- Consider the patient's travel history, as schistosomiasis can cause dysuria, especially around the Nile.
- Vaginal and urethral trauma, including sexual abuse and the insertion of a foreign body, can cause dysuria.
- Consider malignancy. Carcinoma *in situ* of the bladder can present as dysuria.

Urinary incontinence

Overview

The prevalence of urinary incontinence (more than two episodes per month) is 8.5% in women aged 15–64 years, and 11.6% in those over 65 years. This is likely to be an underestimate.

Incontinence can be defined according to the following criteria:

- urge – increase in abdominal pressure
- true – absence of detrusor activity
- overflow – defect of urethral sphincter.

Specific areas for consideration when taking a history

- Duration and occurrence.
- Obstetric history.
- History of:
  - travel
  - irradiation
  - pelvic surgery.

Differential diagnosis

Common	Occasional	Rare
• Following childbirth – mechanical and denervation injury • Post menopause – reduced intra-urethral pressure due to low oestrogen levels	• Chronic UTI • Detrusor instability • Social – impaired access to toilet facilities	• Calculi (rarely associated with incontinence, usually associated with frequency) • True incontinence – communication between ureter or bladder and uterus/vagina (e.g. vesico-vaginal fistula, uretero-vaginalfistula) • Pelvic surgery irradiation • Bladder malignancy • TB • Schistosomiasis

Possible investigations

- Urinalysis – to check for signs of UTI.
- MSU – to confirm infection and guide treatment.
- Pelvic USS – to detect calculi or other masses.
- Cystoscopy, cystometry and contrast radiography – to visualise pathology.
- Tuberculin skin test and chest X-ray – to detect TB.

Notes

- Consider the psychological effects of incontinence. It can have a devastating impact on self-esteem and seriously affect a woman's social and sexual functioning.

Hazard warnings

- Continuous incontinence suggests significant pathology, such as a fistula, chronic outflow obstruction or a neurological problem.

Pregnancy

- **Abdominal pain in pregnancy**

- **Bleeding in pregnancy**

- **Infertility**

Abdominal pain in pregnancy

Overview

Occasional abdominal discomfort is a common complaint in pregnancy, and although it is usually harmless, it can also be a sign of a serious problem.

History

- Duration and type of pain (severe and persistent pain is not normal).
- Associated symptoms (e.g. PV bleeding, vomiting, diarrhoea).
- Previous operations (bowel distortion).
- Medication.

Differential diagnosis

Common	Occasional	Rare
• UTI • Gas and bloating • Dyspepsia • Constipation • Round ligament pain (second trimester) • Braxton Hicks contractions • Back pain	• Ectopic pregnancy (first trimester) • Miscarriage (usually associated with bleeding) • Preterm labour • Placental abruption (late gestation) • Endometriosis • Ovarian cyst • Appendicitis • Virus/food poisoning • Kidney stones • Hepatitis • Gall bladder disease • Pancreatitis • Bowel obstruction	• Pubic symphysis separation • Hepatic rupture (associated with severe pre-eclampsia, close to term) • Degeneration of a uterine myoma (haemorrhagic infarction of a uterine fibroid – rapid, local, severe pain) • Peptic ulcer disease • Mesenteric vein thrombosis

Possible investigations

- Blood pressure – to identify pre-eclampsia.
- Urinalysis:
  - protein to identify pre-eclampsia
  - nitrites to identify UTI.
- MSU – to identify UTI.
- Pelvic examination – to detect pelvic tenderness and possible infection.
- Speculum examination – to facilitate sexual health screen.
- Sexual health screen – to identify specific STIs.
- Serum βHCG – to assess whether pregnancy is growing or failing.
- Sickle screen (to identify presence of sickle cell trait or anaemia).
- USS – to identify cysts, ectopic pregnancy or miscarriage.

Notes

- Anatomical landmarks are shifted by a pregnant uterus.
- Pain on standing and walking that is relieved by rest, with pubic symphysis tenderness, is symphyseal pain and is often overlooked.

Hazard warnings

- Distortion of anatomy may alter symptoms and signs. Appendicitis is notoriously difficult to diagnose in the second trimester. The patient should be referred.
- Consider the possibility of ectopic pregnancy in a woman who experiences unilateral lower abdominal pain in early pregnancy.
- Placental abruption causes severe, continuous pain with a tender, hard uterus. Vaginal bleeding may be minimal. The patient should be admitted immediately.
- Pre-eclampsia may cause epigastric pain in the third trimester.

Bleeding in pregnancy

Overview

Around 10–30% of women experience bleeding in pregnancy with no adverse outcome, especially in the first trimester.

History

- Duration and nature of bleeding, and associated pain.
- Sexual health history.
- Surgical history.
- Congenital abnormalities of the reproductive tract.
- Obstetric history.
- Drug use.

Differential diagnosis

Common	Occasional	Rare
• Implantation bleed, usually 11–12 days after fertilisation	• Spontaneous abortion (miscarriage)	• Polyps
	• Threatened miscarriage	• Cervical cancer
• Trauma and tears to vaginal wall during sexual intercourse	• Completed miscarriage	• Varicose veins
	• Incomplete miscarriage	• Uterine rupture
	• Blighted ovum	• Fetal vessel rupture
• Inflamed cervix due to vaginal infection or STI	• Missed abortion (intrauterine fetal demise, IUFD)	
	• Molar pregnancy (gestational trophoblastic disease)	
	• Placenta praevia	
	• Placental abruption	
	• Ectopic pregnancy (associated with abdominal pain)	
	• Early labour	

Possible investigations

- Urinalysis – to detect possible UTI.
- Blood βHCG and progestogen levels – to assess whether pregnancy is growing or failing.
- Blood type and rhesus status – in acute scenario where additional blood or exchange transfusion is required.
- Pelvic USS – to detect viability of pregnancy, location of a bleed or location of placenta.
- Bimanual examination – may elicit tenderness indicative of an STI.
- Speculum examination – to facilitate sexual health screen.
- Sexual health screen – to identify specific STIs.
- Fetal monitoring – to assess fetal well-being.

Notes

- It is important to distinguish between spotting and bleeding in pregnancy. The former may be due to an increase in the blood supply to the cervix and greater blood flow to the area. Spotting may occur after having a cervical smear, an internal examination, or intercourse.
- If symptoms are acute, bed rest may be recommended. Little research has been carried out, but to date it has not shown bed rest to be helpful. It is important that the woman's preferences with regard to bed rest are taken into consideration.
- Avoidance of sexual intercourse is advised during any period of vaginal bleeding. Some authors recommend that sexual intercourse should be avoided for 2 to 3 weeks after the bleeding has settled.

Hazard warnings

- The amount of bleeding is proportional to the risk of miscarriage the heavier the bleeding, the higher the risk of miscarriage. Abdominal pain associated with the bleeding is not considered to be a good sign.
- Unilateral pelvic pain with vaginal bleeding within 2 weeks of a missed period suggests an ectopic pregnancy, and the patient should be referred immediately.

Infertility

Overview

One in seven couples now has trouble conceiving naturally. In approximately 30% of infertile couples the cause is identified only in the female, and in 30% the cause is identified only in the male. In 30% of couples, causes can be detected in both partners. In about 10% of cases the underlying cause is not found by current diagnostic methods.

History

- Duration of infertility.
- Menstrual history.
- Medication.
- Contraception history.
- Obstetric history.
- Surgical history.
- Family history of chromosomal disorders.
- Medical history (e.g. childhood malignancy).
- BMI.

Differential diagnosis

Common	Occasional	Rare
• Age • Weight • Exercise • PCOS • Pelvic infection (e.g. chlamydia, PID) • Endometriosis	• Medication • Hyperprolactinaemia • Hypogonadotrophic hypogonadism • Hypopituitarism • Premature ovarian failure • IDDM-related sexual dysfunction • Psychological loss of libido	• Surgical cause • Mucus hostility – antisperm antibodies • Increased mucus viscosity • Male factor: Obstructive azoospermia Severe sperm dysfunction Primary testicular failure Congenital abnormality Post chemotherapy/ radiotherapy Endocrine disturbance

Possible investigations

- Serum hormone levels (FSH, LH, prolactin, testosterone and oestrogen) – to confirm ovulation.
- Pelvic examination – to check the mobility of the pelvic organs.
- Speculum examination – to facilitate sexual health screen.
- Sexual health screen – to identify specific STIs.
- Post-coital test for sperm–mucus interaction.
- Hysterosalpingogram – to identify tubal blockage.
- Contrast ultrasonography – to identify tubal blockage.
- Laparoscopy – to identify pathology, or for possible removal of adhesions.
- Hysteroscopy – to identify fibroids, septae, adhesions and polyps.

Notes

- Infertility can be caused by lifestyle factors such as stress, smoking, alcohol, obesity and STIs.
- Counselling with regard to fertile times in the menstrual cycle may be useful.
- Women who are actively trying to become pregnant should receive pre-conception advice about diet, alcohol, smoking, rubella status and folic acid.

Hazard warnings

- Infertility is rarely the presenting problem of serious pathology. However, there are circumstances in which it is important to refer the patient immediately – if the woman is over 35 years of age, has amenorrhoea, has a history of pelvic surgery or PID, or has any abnormality on pelvic examination.

Weight

- **Weight gain**

- **Weight loss**

Weight gain

Overview

Weight gain is more likely to affect women between the ages of 35 and 55 years. During this time, weight can be gained, or maintaining a steady weight becomes more difficult.

Weight gain can have serious implications for health. Excess weight can increase the risk of the following:

- high cholesterol
- high blood pressure
- insulin resistance, which can lead to type 2 diabetes.

All of these factors can increase the risk of heart disease.

History

- Familial tendency.
- Dietary history.
- Lifestyle.
- Life events/stress.
- Menstrual history.
- Obstetric history.

Differential diagnosis

Common	Occasional	Rare
• Overeating (e.g. comfort eating due to stress)	• Depression	• Cushing's syndrome
	• Genetic tendency	• Prader–Willi syndrome
• Pregnancy	• Ovarian cyst	• Laurence–Moon–Biedl syndrome
• Recent childbirth	• Hypothyroidism	
• Depressive disorders	• Causes of oedema (PMS, heart failure, kidney conditions, liver conditions)	• Brain disorder causing overeating
• Sedentary lifestyle/ lack of exercise		
• Giving up smoking	• Medication (e.g. combined oral contraceptive/HRT, psychotropic drugs, corticosteroids, antiretrovirals, thiazolidinediones)	
• Menopause		
• PCOS		
• Hypoglycaemia	• Hormonal contraception (e.g. Depo-Provera injection)	

Possible investigations

- Urinary βHCG – to detect pregnancy.
- Blood tests – TFTs, U&Es and hormone levels to detect liver or thyroid problems and PCOS.
- Genetic screen – to detect syndromes.
- Pelvic USS – to detect PCOS, cysts, etc.

Notes

- Exercise and dietary advice are essential.

Hazard warnings

Establish whether the weight gain is diffuse or predominantly abdominal. The latter may indicate pregnancy, ascites or a large ovarian cyst.

Weight loss

Overview

Weight loss is a non-specific symptom. Acute weight loss could indicate underlying pathology. In about one-third of cases there is no specific cause. Of the remainder, some have psychiatric causes and 90% are due to organic illness.

History

- General and medication history.
- Dietary history.

- Exercise.
- Lifestyle (including drug use).
- Life events.
- Psychological assessment.

Differential diagnosis

Common	Occasional	Rare
• Poor diet	• Depression	• Stomach/colon cancer
• Increase in exercise	• Grief	• Oesophageal carcinoma
• Dieting	• Alcohol/drug abuse	• Oesophageal reflux
• Anxiety	• Hiatus hernia	• Thyrotoxicosis
	• Chronic pancreatitis	• HIV
	• Coeliac disease	• Parkinson's disease
	• Crohn's disease	• Alzheimer's disease
	• Ulcerative colitis	• Anorexia nervosa
	• Diabetes	
	• Hyperthyroidism	
	• Stomach cancer	
	• Stomach ulcer	
	• Side-effects of certain drugs and sedatives (e.g. NSAIDs)	

Possible investigations

- Blood tests:
  - FBC and ESR – haemoglobin may be reduced and ESR may be elevated in malignancy and any chronic disorder
  - U&Es – abnormal in renal failure and sometimes in eating disorders
  - TFTs – to confirm hyperthyroidism.
- Sexual health screen – to detect STIs, notably HIV.
- Tests to exclude malignancy, which include the following:
  - barium meal
  - faecal occult blood test
  - ultrasound
  - X-ray
  - CT scan
  - endoscopy/colonoscopy
  - biopsy.

Notes

- Establish whether there has actually been any weight loss. There may be a measurement from previous encounters with which to compare the current measurement.

Hazard warnings

- Rapid weight loss with malaise and respiratory or gastrointestinal symptoms strongly suggests a physical cause.
- Consider eating disorders in girls and young women.

Conditions

Pregnancy

- **Blighted ovum**

- **Braxton Hicks contractions**

- **Early labour**

- **Ectopic pregnancy**

- **Miscarriage**

- **Molar pregnancy**

- **Placental abruption**

- **Placenta praevia**

- **Postnatal depression**

- **Pre-eclampsia**

- **Preterm labour**

- **Pubic symphysis separation**

- **Round ligament pain**

Blighted ovum

A blighted ovum is a fertilised egg that has ceased development at a very early stage. On ultrasound examination there is a gestational sac in which no fetal pole can be identified. Because the egg's supporting tissue (trophoblast) may continue to function for some time after the death of the embryo, the sac may reach a considerable size.

A blighted ovum is an example of a spontaneous abortion. Spontaneous abortion occurs in 15% of human pregnancies, with most occurring during the first trimester. In more than half of spontaneous abortions there are abnormal chromosomes. Although small studies suggest that enzyme deficiencies in placental tissues or abnormal expression of genes on particular chromosomes may be responsible for some cases of blighted ovum, the causes are likely to be similar to the causes of spontaneous abortion in general.

Expectant management or conservative management involves no action being taken and the woman miscarries naturally. This may take some time. Alternatively, the woman can undergo an operation to remove the blighted ovum (evacuation of retained products of conception, ERPC). Some centres use medication to initiate contractions and soften the cervix to allow the retained products of conception to pass.

Resources

www.womens-health.co.uk/blighted.html
www.miscarriageassociation.org.uk/ma2006/information/leaflets/why.pdf

Braxton Hicks contractions

Named after John Braxton Hicks (1823–1897), a British gynaecologist, these are irregular contractions of the womb that occur towards the middle of pregnancy in the first pregnancy, and earlier and more intensely in subsequent pregnancies. These contractions tend to occur during physical activity. The uterus tightens for 30 to 60 seconds, beginning at the top of the uterus, and the contraction gradually spreads downward before the uterus relaxes. Although they are said to be painless, Braxton Hicks contractions may be quite uncomfortable and are sometimes difficult to distinguish from the contractions of true labour.

Early labour

Labour that takes place before 37 weeks is considered to be premature. Infants who are born as a result of premature labour suffer significant morbidity as a result of immaturity. Accurate diagnosis of preterm labour can allow for the prevention or delay of preterm birth where possible, and where this is not possible, earlier provision can be made to provide optimal support for the immature infant.

Many factors are now known to increase the risk of premature labour, including the following:

- previous premature labour
- multiple pregnancy
- prolonged bleeding in early pregnancy
- maternal cardiac disease
- maternal age < 15 years
- cigarette smoking during pregnancy
- low BMI
- cervical incompetence
- infection (e.g. chorioamnionitis, bacterial vaginosis)
- low social class
- unsupported and/or single mothers.

Babies who are delivered with optimal care after 30 weeks most often survive without any lasting abnormality. Babies who are delivered before 26 weeks have an increased risk of long-term disability. Babies born at 23–24 weeks' gestation have a 50% risk of lasting disability.

Ectopic pregnancy

An ectopic pregnancy occurs when a fertilised egg attaches itself outside the cavity of the uterus. The majority of ectopic pregnancies are found in the uterine tubes. In rare cases, the egg attaches itself within one of the ovaries, the cervix or another organ within the pelvis.

The most common symptoms and findings of ectopic pregnancy are as follows:

- an overdue period (suggesting pregnancy)
- bleeding from the vagina
- a positive pregnancy test
- lower abdominal pain
- fainting.

At first an ectopic pregnancy develops like a normal pregnancy and the same symptoms, such as nausea and breast tenderness, will be present. However, some women do not have these symptoms and do not suspect that they are pregnant. If a woman is pregnant and has long-lasting throbbing in one side of the lower abdomen, or if she is experiencing sudden pain, a referral to an acute gynaecology service is required, as an ectopic pregnancy can be life-threatening if it ruptures and causes internal bleeding.

Risk factors may be present that increase the likelihood of a woman experiencing an ectopic pregnancy. These include the following:

- previous surgery to the uterine tubes or previous inflammation of the uterine tubes (PID). As the lining of the tubes is so delicate, inflammation or trauma can cause the cilia to beat in an abnormal fashion so that the fertilised egg implants in the wrong place
- previous ectopic pregnancy. If there has been a previous ectopic pregnancy, the chances of another one occurring are increased
- becoming pregnant while using a contraceptive IUD or the progestogen-only contraceptive pill (mini-pill)
- becoming pregnant through IVF. One or more eggs are inserted into the woman's uterus. Despite being placed within the womb, the fertilised egg may still attach itself to the wrong area outside the cavity of the uterus
- many women who experience an ectopic pregnancy do not have any of these risk factors.

Diagnosis

- A urine test for pregnancy. In cases of doubt, a blood pregnancy test may be performed, which is always positive in ectopic pregnancy.
- In the case of ectopic pregnancy, the uterus will often be smaller than expected for the number of weeks since the woman's last period. This can be checked by an internal pelvic examination. The clinician might feel a tender swelling corresponding to an ectopic pregnancy.

- An ultrasound scan will help the clinician to differentiate between a possible miscarriage, a continuing pregnancy inside the womb and an ectopic pregnancy.
- Further investigation depends on the woman's symptoms, the scan findings and the level of pregnancy hormone (βHCG) in the woman's blood. If there is uncertainty about the diagnosis, waiting for 48 hours and then measuring the level of βHCG again is often appropriate.

Treatment

If an ectopic pregnancy is strongly suspected, the gynaecologist will perform a laparoscopy to confirm the diagnosis. Laparoscopy is performed through small incisions in the abdominal wall, and the ectopic pregnancy can usually be removed via this route. The uterine tube in which the ectopic pregnancy occurred is often, but not always, removed at the same time. In some instances, open surgery becomes necessary, with the pregnancy being removed through a larger incision above the pubic hair line.

An alternative treatment to surgery is a medicine called methotrexate, which decreases the growth of cells in the ectopic pregnancy (unlicensed use). As a result the pregnancy shrinks and eventually disappears. The advantage of methotrexate is that it avoids the need for surgery, but success rates with this drug tend to be slightly lower than with surgery. Occasionally, both surgery and methotrexate will be necessary.

Future pregnancy

The outlook for future pregnancies depends on several factors, especially whether the other uterine tube appeared normal or not. As a general guide, after one ectopic pregnancy, 20% of women will experience another ectopic pregnancy, 30% will not become pregnant again and 50% will have a successful pregnancy inside the womb.

Resources

www.ectopic.org
www.womens-health.co.uk/ectopic.asp
www.miscarriageassociation.org.uk/ma2006/information/leaflets/ectopic.pdf

Miscarriage

Miscarriage is the spontaneous discharge of the gestation sac before the fetus is viable. The term applies to losses up to 24 weeks. Spontaneous miscarriage occurs in about 50% of pregnancies, 15% of which are clinically recognised. The vast majority occur in the first 14 days following conception. Increasing maternal age is associated with increased fetal loss.

Threatened miscarriage is the earliest stage of most spontaneous miscarriages. There is bleeding from the genital tract, but the cervix is closed and there is no discharge of products of conception. Inevitable spontaneous miscarriage occurs in about 25% of women with a threatened miscarriage.

A complete, incomplete or missed miscarriage may result.

Incomplete miscarriage

In an incomplete miscarriage, the products of conception have not been completely lost from the uterus. It is most likely to occur between 8 and 14 weeks' gestation, when the placenta is not expelled completely and an evacuation of the retained products of conception (ERPC) is necessary.

Complete miscarriage

In a complete miscarriage, all the products of conception have been lost from the uterus. This is most likely to occur before 8 weeks' gestation, and an ERPC may not be necessary.

Missed miscarriage

In a missed miscarriage, there is fetal death before 24 weeks' gestation, but the fetus is not lost from the uterus.

Diagnosis

Fetal heartbeat is absent on ultrasound.

First-trimester abortions are rarely recurrent. They should therefore only be investigated after three or more miscarriages. Second-trimester abortions are much rarer and more likely to recur, and should therefore be investigated fully.

Resources

www.womens-health.co.uk/miscarr.htm
www.miscarriageassociation.org.uk

Molar pregnancy

This is a benign tumour arising from the trophoblast, and it occurs in 1 in 2,500 to 1 in 5,000 pregnancies in the UK. Pathologically, a 'hydatidiform mole' or molar pregnancy appears as a mass of vesicles that is classically described as a 'bunch of grapes.' Complete moles are characterised by extensive proliferation of trophoblastic tissue, hydropic villi and the absence of fetal vessels. In an incomplete mole, overgrowth of trophoblastic tissue is less marked, some villi are normal and fetal vessels are present. In a molar pregnancy, βHCG levels are raised. About 2% of moles develop into choriocarcinomas.

Hydatidiform mole is usually suspected on the basis of the clinical picture, namely bleeding after a prolonged period of amenorrhoea, early pre-eclampsia, excessive vomiting with the pregnancy, or (in 50% of cases) a uterus which is large for dates.

Diagnosis

- Examination for hydropic villi in vaginal blood.
- Serum βHCG levels – usually high for early pregnancy.
- USS – characteristic 'snowstorm' pattern.

Treatment

- Suction evacuation.
- Arrange for weekly monitoring of βHCG levels to detect recurrence.
- Chemotherapy may be indicated if metastasis is detected.

Further treatment

- Monitor βHCG levels 2- to 4-weekly for the next 1–2 years.
- Avoid pregnancy until βHCG levels have returned to normal.
- For an incomplete mole, evacuation is rarely needed, as spontaneous termination of the pregnancy tends to precede detection of the mole. Importantly, partial moles are not reported to metastasise, so chemotherapy is rarely required.

Resources

www.hmole-chorio.org.uk
www.miscarriageassociation.org.uk/ma2006/information/leaflets/hydamole.htm

Placental abruption

Separation of the placenta from its uterine attachment results in a maternal bleed from the opened sinuses. The clinical features of placental abruption depend on the size and site of the bleeding. A bleed which tracks down behind the membranes and appears through the cervix is said to be 'revealed', whereas a bleed that occurs retroplacentally is said to be 'concealed.'

In extreme cases, profuse abruption, pain, shock, uterine rigidity and absent fetal heart sounds are evident. In milder cases, the following symptoms and signs may occur singly or in combination, or none of them may be present:

- vaginal bleeding
- uterine tenderness and back pain
- fetal distress
- high-frequency uterine contractions of low tone
- idiopathic preterm labour
- hypotension leading to rapid shock.

Mild abruption requires a short stay in hospital, with the patient then being discharged if there is no recurrence of bleeding. Moderate abruption requires hospitalisation and monitoring with induction at term. Severe abruption requires obstetric emergency care with delivery by Caesarean section. If the fetus is no longer viable, a vaginal delivery is medically preferable.

Placenta praevia

Placenta praevia is said to occur when a placenta is situated in the lower uterine segment. There are varying degrees of abnormality associated with an increasing need for a Caesarean section instead of a spontaneous vaginal delivery. Placenta praevia occurs in about 0.5% of pregnancies.

Placenta praevia is not inevitable after low implantation, and ultrasound examination has shown that the majority of such cases either abort or resolve as the uterus grows. A large placenta can causes placenta praevia, as its lower portion completely or partially overlaps the internal os. Atrophy and inflammation, perhaps secondary to previous Caesarean section, cause defective decidual vascularisation and hence placenta praevia. Placenta praevia is not usually dangerous for the mother or the baby. However, postpartum haemorrhage is more common with placenta praevia because of the reduced ability of the lower segment to retract.

Diagnosis

Placenta praevia usually occurs after 30 weeks' gestation. It presents with recurrent, painless vaginal bleeding. A vaginal examination should not be performed, as severe haemorrhage may be provoked by disturbing the blood vessels that lie across the os. History and examination are the main tools for diagnosis, and USS can improve diagnostic accuracy.

Treatment

Bed rest and hospitalisation are advised in order to try to ensure that the pregnancy goes to term. A Caesarean section may be indicated.

Postnatal depression

Postnatal depression is defined as depression that occurs within 12 months of childbirth.

There are three main types of postnatal depression:

- postpartum blues
- depressive illness
- puerperal psychosis.

Postpartum blues

Postpartum blues is a mild disturbance in mood that occurs within 1 week of delivery. Its incidence is estimated to be 50–70%, and it is more common following the birth of a first child. The usual features include crying, fatigue, sensitivity to criticism, anxiety, irritability, helplessness and lability of mood. Symptoms last from a few hours to a few days.

Depressive illness

The peak incidence of depressive illness appears to occur at 3 months, but with significant numbers of cases still appearing by 6 months or later. Depressive illness occurs after 10–15% of pregnancies. The usual features are similar to those of non-psychotic depression appearing in women at any other time of life.

Puerperal psychosis

Puerperal psychosis is a rare complication of childbirth, with an incidence of about 1 to 2 per 1,000 births. The onset is usually 2 to 4 days after delivery, and the condition is often characterised by clouding of consciousness, perplexity, delusions and hallucinations. Paranoid delusions often centre around the child. Consequently, there may be a risk of infanticide or injury to the child. Apart from this specific risk, the child may suffer neglect or inappropriate treatment at the hands of a psychotic mother. Treatment of puerperal psychosis usually involves admission of the mother to hospital, preferably with the baby. In this setting the relationship between mother and baby can be preserved without putting the baby at risk. Electroconvulsive therapy (ECT) may be necessary together with tranquillisers, practical help with the child, and support for the rest of the family.

Resources

www.mind.org.uk/Information/Booklets/Understanding/Understanding+postnatal+depression.htm
www.pni.org.uk

Pre-eclampsia

Pre-eclampsia is defined as pregnancy-induced high blood pressure and elimination of protein in the urine. Mild pre-eclampsia occurs in 1 in 10 mothers, is severe in 1 in 50, and progresses to eclampsia in 1 in 3,500. Pre-eclampsia is a major cause of intrauterine growth retardation and perinatal mortality. Typically, pre-eclampsia occurs after 20 weeks' gestation.

Poor placental perfusion causes the release of bloodborne products from the feto-placental unit, which result in endothelial cell dysfunction. There is an increased sensitivity to normal circulating pressor agents, increased intracellular coagulation and increased fluid loss from the intravascular compartment.

Causes of a poorly perfused placenta include the following:

- abnormal trophoblast implantation and spiral artery atherosis
- microvascular disease – pre-existing hypertension, diabetes, collagen vascular diseases
- a large placenta – multiple pregnancy, hydatidiform mole, a fetus with a hydropic placenta.

Pre-eclampsia is more common in first pregnancies and in women whose mothers or sisters had pre-eclampsia. The risk of pre-eclampsia is higher in women carrying multiple babies, in teenage mothers and in women over 40 years of age. Other women at risk include those who had high blood pressure or kidney disease before they became pregnant. The exact cause of pre-eclampsia is not known.

The only cure for pre-eclampsia is to stop the pregnancy and deliver the placenta despite the possible risk to the fetus. This will require careful consideration of hospital admission, timing of the delivery, the control of established disease with antihypertensive and anticonvulsant therapy, and disease prevention (e.g. by means of aspirin and diet).

Preterm labour

Preterm labour is defined as labour that occurs before 37 weeks' gestation. Premature onset of labour may occur spontaneously or it may be induced for therapeutic reasons.

Natural causes of premature birth include the following:

- 50% unknown
- multiple pregnancy – typically for twins delivery occurs between 36 and 38 weeks, and for triplets it occurs at around 32 weeks
- polyhydramnios (excessive amniotic fluid)
- cervical incompetence and uterine anomalies
- premature rupture of membranes – 30–40% of cases start labour within 24 hours of the rupture
- intrauterine infection
- maternal malnutrition
- maternal infection.

Premature birth may be iatrogenically induced for a variety of reasons, including:

- pregnancy-induced proteinuric hypertension (e.g. pre-eclampsia or eclampsia)
- maternal renal disease or cardiac disease
- intrauterine infection, particularly after premature rupture of membranes
- antepartum haemorrhage
- intrauterine growth retardation.

Gestational age is the single most important prognostic factor when assessing the effects of prematurity. The lower the gestational age, the higher the risk of morbidity and mortality.

Pubic symphysis separation

Pubic symphysis separation is a recognised complication of pregnancy, and its incidence has been estimated to range from 1 in 300 to 1 in 30,000. Characteristic symptoms of symphyseal separation include suprapubic pain and tenderness with radiation to the back of the legs, difficulty in walking and (occasionally) bladder dysfunction. The cause is not fully understood, but there may be a genetic pre-disposition. There are also associations with multiparity, large babies, pathology of the joints (causing loosening) and increased force placed on the pelvic ring.

Diagnosis

Diagnosis of symphyseal separation can be made on the basis of history alone, but X-ray and USS are frequently used to confirm the diagnosis. Trauma or obstetric interventions such as application of force to move the thighs or the use of forceps may also trigger separation.

Postpartum signs may include urinary incontinence when changing position from supine or prone to upright, pain in the hips or lower back when walking, or a waddling gait when walking. The change in gait and the pain when walking may not be noticed until 24 hours or more after delivery.

Treatment

Treatment is usually conservative, including bed rest, pelvic binders, the use of walkers and mild analgesics, which usually results in complete recovery within 4 to 6 weeks. The occurrence of a symphyseal separation should not significantly alter the management of subsequent pregnancies, and the same types of con-servative therapy are recommended for any recurrence of symptoms. Recurrent separation of the symphysis pubis could occur during subsequent deliveries, but generally is no worse than the first occurrence.

Round ligament pain

Round ligaments on either side of the uterus attach it to the abdomen and hold it in place. During pregnancy, the uterus enlarges to make room for the growing baby. This puts strain on the round ligaments and may cause pain. The problem is not serious and is a normal part of pregnancy.

Pelvic conditions

- Bartholinitis

- Cervical cancer

- Cervical incompetence

- Ectropion

- Endometriosis and adenomyosis

- Fibroids

- Ovarian cyst

- Ovulation pain

- Pelvic/vulval abscess

- Pelvic congestion

- Pelvic fistula

- Pelvic inflammatory disease

- Pelvic organ prolapse

- Polycystic ovarian syndrome

- Polyps

- Pyometra

- Vaginismus

- Vulval intra-epithelial neoplasia

- Vulval tuberculosis

Female reproductive organs

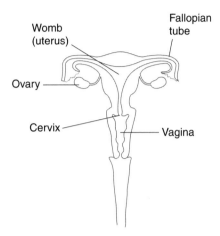

Figure 1   Female reproductive organs: front view.

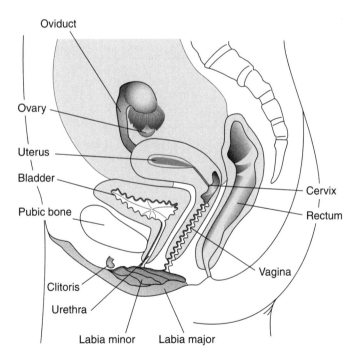

Figure 2   Female reproductive organs: side view.

Bartholinitis

This is a common benign lesion of the vulva, involving a dilatation of the duct of Bartholin's gland. It typically presents as a unilateral swelling on the postero-lateral aspect of the introitus. The cyst is usually about 2 cm in diameter but may be up to 8 cm. It contains sterile mucus and is asymptomatic.

Secondary infection of the cyst produces a Bartholin's abscess, which is often tender. Treatment is by marsupialisation of the gland to create a fistulous tract between the wall of the duct and the skin.

Recurrent infection in older women should raise the rare possibility of carcinoma.

Cervical cancer

There are two main types of cervical cancer. The most common type is *squamous-cell carcinoma*, which develops from the flat cells that cover the outer surface of the cervix at the top of the vagina (the transformation zone). The other type is *adenocarcinoma*, which develops from the glandular cells that line the cervical canal (endocervix). As adenocarcinoma starts in the cervical canal, it may be more difficult to detect with cervical screening tests. There are other less common types of cancer of the cervix, known as *adenosquamous carcinoma*, and *clear-cell* and *small-cell carcinoma*.

Symptoms

- Abnormal vaginal bleeding (e.g. between periods or after intercourse).
- Malodorous vaginal discharge.
- Discomfort during intercourse.
- In post-menopausal women there may be new bleeding.

Prevalence

Cervical cancer is the eleventh commonest cause of cancer deaths in women in the UK, accounting for around 2% of all female cancers. The incidence of cervical cancer fell by 42% between 1988 and 1997 in England and Wales. This decrease is directly related to the cervical screening programme.

Cervical screening programme

In women under the age of 25 years, invasive cancer is extremely rare, but changes in the cervix are common. In the UK, women currently receive their first invitation for cervical screening at the age of 25 years. Three-yearly screening is recommended between the ages of 25 and 49 years. Between the ages of 50 and 64 years, 5-yearly screening is recommended. From the age of 65 years onwards only those women who have not been screened since the age of 50 or who have had recent abnormal tests should be screened.

Diagnosis

- Smear test.
- Liquid-based cytology.
- Colposcopy.

Smear test

The smear test involves inserting a plastic or metal speculum into the vagina to hold the walls of the vagina open, so that the neck of the womb/cervix can be seen. A wooden or plastic spatula and/or a specially shaped brush is then stroked around the cervix. Some cells from the surface of the cervix become attached to the spatula or brush. These are then smeared on to a glass slide, which is treated with alcohol to preserve the cells, and sent to a special cytology laboratory to be examined under a microscope.

This form of testing is now becoming less frequent, as liquid-based cytology is a more accurate form of testing, although there are some clinical situations where a cervical smear may still be preferred (e.g. in a pregnant woman with HIV).

Liquid-based cytology

The sample is collected in a similar way to the smear test, using a spatula which brushes cells from the neck of the womb. The head of the spatula, where the cells are lodged, is broken off into a small vial containing preservative fluid, or rinsed directly into the preservative fluid. The sample is then sent to the laboratory, where it is centrifuged and treated to remove obscuring material (e.g. mucus, pus), and a random sample of the remaining cells is taken. A thin layer of cells is deposited on to a slide, which is then examined under a microscope by a cytologist.

Coloposcopy

If a woman has had an abnormal cervical smear, it is necessary to examine her cervix with a special microsocope called a colposcope. The woman sits on a couch which supports her legs, and a speculum is passed to visualise the cervix (just like having a smear).

To identify the site, grade and shape of the abnormal area of cells, the clinician who is performing the colposcopy examination will stain the cervix in the area of the transformation zone.

A solution of acetic acid is then gently wiped on the cervix. Abnormal dyskaryotic/dysplastic cells will stain white and, as a general rule, the more dense the white area becomes, the higher the grade of abnormality.

A water-based solution of iodine is then gently applied to the rest of the cervix to identify the complete area of abnormality. Iodine stains the normal cells black and the abnormal cells yellow.

In most cases there is a good correlation between the abnormality suggested by the cervical smear and the appearance as seen through the colposcope. A small biopsy can be taken for analysis. This is done using special biopsy forceps to remove a small fragment of tissue with minimal discomfort to the patient.

Staging

The *stage* of a cancer describes its size and whether it has spread beyond its original site. Knowing the extent of the cancer and the grade helps to determine the most appropriate treatment.

The stages of cervical cancer are described below.

- *Stage 1.* The cancer cells are confined to the cervix.
- *Stage 2.* The tumour has spread into surrounding structures such as the upper part of the vagina or the tissues adjacent to the cervix.
- *Stage 3.* The tumour has spread to surrounding structures such as the lower part of the vagina, nearby lymph nodes, or tissues at the sides of the pelvic area.
- *Stage 4.* The tumour has spread to the bladder or bowel or beyond the pelvic area. This stage includes tumours that have spread into the lungs, liver or bone, although these are not common.

Grading

Grading refers to the appearance of the cancer cells under the microscope. The grade gives an idea of how quickly the cancer may develop. There are three grades: grade 1 (low grade), grade 2 (moderate grade) and grade 3 (high grade). In low-grade tumours the cancer cells look very like the normal cells of the cervix. These tumours are usually slow-growing and less likely to spread. In high-grade tumours the cells look very abnormal. These tumours are likely to grow more quickly and are more likely to spread.

Treatment

Large loop excision of the transformation zone (LLETZ)

LLETZ is used to remove the area of the cervix that contains the abnormal cells, which can then be examined under a microscope in the laboratory. LLETZ is usually performed under local anaesthetic, and a thin wire is used to cut away the affected area.

Cone biopsy

If the abnormal area cannot be seen properly with the colposcope, a cone biopsy may be performed. A small cone-shaped section of the cervix, large enough to remove any abnormal cells, is taken for examination under a microscope by a pathologist. If there is only a very small growth of cancer cells, the cone biopsy may remove it all so that no further treatment is needed. If the cancer is more developed and the cone biopsy has not removed all of the cancer cells, it is still helpful for determining the diagnosis and treatment pathways.

Surgery

Surgery is often the main treatment for cancer of the cervix in its early stages (where it is confined to the cervix).

Radiotherapy

Radiotherapy is as effective as surgery in this situation, but the side-effects are more severe. For this reason, surgery is usually used. Radiotherapy is sometimes used after surgery if there is a risk that some cancer cells may have been left behind, to help to reduce the risk of the cancer recurring. Sometimes radiotherapy is combined with chemotherapy – this is known as concomitant therapy or chemoradiotherapy.

Chemotherapy

Chemotherapy is occasionally used before surgery in order to shrink the cancer and make the operation easier, but it is mainly given with radiotherapy after surgery.

Resources

www.cancerscreening.nhs.uk/cervical/index.html
www.cancerbacup.org.uk/Cancertype/Cervix
National Cervical Cancer Coalition; www.nccc-online.org
www.colposcopy.org.uk

Cervical incompetence

Cervical incompetence occurs when the cervix is abnormally prone to dilation during the second trimester of pregnancy, resulting in spontaneous abortion of the fetus. Evacuation is usually painless and without associated bleeding. Uterine contractions are uncommon.

Cervical incompetence is congenital in up to 30% of women in whom the uterus has a congenital fundal abnormality, or may result from exposure to diethyl-stilboestrol *in utero*.

However, the vast majority of cases are acquired, most frequently as a result of trauma. For example:

- lateral cervical tears at the time of delivery
- cone biopsy for investigation of malignancy
- surgical dilation and evacuation for termination of pregnancy, especially if dilated beyond 8–10 mm.

Uncommonly, incompetence may be attributed to hormonal activity in pregnancy (the normal non-pregnant cervix may become incompetent as hormonal activity causes relaxation), to high collagenolytic activity (producing a weak and distensible cervix), or to a low collagen-to-muscle ratio (the muscle excess compromising sphincter action).

Cervical incompetence may be corrected by cervical encirclage – that is, the placement of a circumferential suture in the supravaginal cervix at the level of the internal os.

A transvaginal approach is most common, with either a Shirodkar or a McDonald suture inserted under general anaesthesia. The Shirodkar suture is placed circumferentially and submucosally, whereas the McDonald suture is inserted without incising the epithelium, and surfaces at the four points of the compass. Each may be tied anteriorly or posteriorly.

Both types of suture are best inserted at 14–16 weeks' gestation. This avoids first-trimester abortions, for which both methods are unhelpful, and precedes cervical effacement and dilation. Both are removed at 38 weeks or earlier if the patient goes into premature labour.

Resources

www.womens-health.co.uk/cxinc.asp
www.nct.org.uk/info/Cervical_Incompetence

Ectropion

This is a condition in which columnar epithelium, continuous from the cervical canal, replaces the stratified squamous epithelium that normally covers the vaginal portion of the cervix. Most patients are asymptomatic except for some mucoid discharge, although there may be some pain and/or bleeding. The diagnosis is confirmed by speculum examination. A cervical smear test should be performed with colposcopy and biopsy as appropriate. A troublesome erosion may be treated by thermal cautery with diathermy, cryosurgery or laser treatment.

Endometriosis and adenomyosis

Endometriosis is a condition in which the cells that are normally found lining the uterus are also found in other areas of the body, usually within the pelvis. Each month this tissue outside the uterus, under normal hormonal control, is built up and then breaks down and bleeds in the same way as the lining of the uterus. This internal bleeding into the pelvis, unlike a period, has no way of leaving the body. This leads to inflammation, pain and the formation of scar tissue. Endometrial tissue can also be found in the ovary, where it may form cysts known as 'chocolate' cysts.

Endometrial tissue can also be found in the muscle layer of the wall of the uterus. This is known as adenomyosis. Each month this tissue within the muscle wall bleeds in the same way as the endometrial tissue in the pelvis. Adenomyosis can also be found in the muscle layer of the perineum.

Endometrial deposits can also be found in more remote sites than the pelvis in or on the bowel, in or on the bladder, in operation scars and in the lungs.

The cause of endometriosis is not known, but several theories have been put forward, including the following:

- retrograde menstruation
- lymphatic or circulatory spread
- genetic predisposition to the condition
- immune dysfunction
- environmental causes, such as dioxin exposure.

The most widely accepted theory is retrograde menstruation. According to this theory, some of the menstrual blood flows backwards down the uterine tubes and into the pelvis. Some of the endometrial cells contained in the menstrual fluid implant on the reproductive organs or other areas in the pelvis, and these implanted cells cause endometriosis. It is not known why these endometrial cells implant in some women and not in others.

Symptoms

The more common symptoms of endometriosis include the following:

- painful and/or heavy periods
- painful sex
- infertility
- fatigue
- problems when opening the bowels.

Other symptoms can include the following:

- painful periods
- pain starting before periods
- pain during or after sexual intercourse
- ovulation pain
- pain on internal examination
- heavy periods with or without clots
- prolonged bleeding
- premenstrual spotting
- irregular periods
- loss of dark or old blood before a period or at the end of a period
- painful bowel movement
- pain before or after opening the bowels
- bleeding from the bowel
- pain when passing urine
- pain before or after passing urine
- symptoms of an irritable bowel – diarrhoea, constipation, colic
- lethargy
- extreme tiredness.

Diagnosis

Laparoscopy and laparotomy.

Treatment

There is a range of treatments for endometriosis, but none of them offer a complete cure. Treatments aim to:

- relieve pain symptoms
- shrink or slow endometrial growth

- preserve or restore fertility
- prevent/delay recurrence of the disease.

Hormonal treatments

Hormonal treatment aims to stop ovulation and allow the endometrial deposits to regress and die. The treatment puts the woman into a pseudo-pregnancy or pseudo-menopause. These hormonal drugs include testosterone derivatives, progestogens, GnRH analogues, the combined oral contraceptive pill, the Mirena coil and Depo-Provera. All of the drugs except the oral contraceptive pill and the Mirena coil have been shown in clinical trials to be equally effective as treatments for endometriosis.

Surgery

Conservative surgery seeks to remove and destroy the endometrial growths. This is done by either laparoscopy or laparotomy. Radical surgery may be necessary in women with severe endometriosis. Hysterectomy can be performed with or without removal of the ovaries. If the ovaries are left in place, the likelihood of persistent disease is increased, with some women needing a further operation to remove the ovaries at a later date. For radical surgery to offer hope of a cure for endometriosis, hysterectomy, removal of the ovaries and removal of any endometrial growths should be undertaken. Radical surgery should be the 'last-resort' treatment and not contemplated until all other treatments have been tried or ruled out.

Resources

www.endometriosis.org
www.endometriosisassn.org
www.endo.org.uk
www.endometriosis.org.uk

Fibroids

Uterine fibroids are benign growths of the uterine muscle, and occur in 30–40% of women. Most fibroids do not cause any problems and do not require treatment. However, some fibroids can cause heavy periods which may lead to anaemia and debilitation. If the fibroids grow large they can give rise to 'compression syndrome', in which adjacent organs such as the bladder and the bowel may be compressed, leading to frequency of urination or constipation and bloating. Compression syndrome may also cause backache and sciatica.

Types of fibroid

- *Submucous fibroids* occur just below the lining of the uterus and can cause menstrual problems, including pain as they grow and move around the pelvic area.

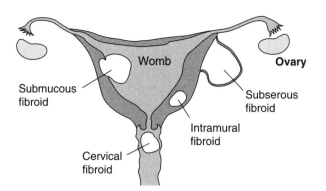

Figure 3 Types of fibroid.

- *Intramural fibroids* are round fibroids, which most often occur within the uterine wall and can cause enlargement of the uterus as they grow.
- *Subserous fibroids* grow on the outer wall of the uterus and usually cause no symptoms until they have become large enough to interfere with other organs.
- *Pedunculated fibroids* develop when a subserous fibroid grows a peduncle (stalk). As they grow larger they may become twisted and cause severe pain.
- *Inter-ligamentous fibroids* grow sideways between the ligaments which support the uterus in the abdominal region. This type of fibroid is especially difficult to remove without interfering with the blood supply of other organs.
- *Parasitic fibroids* are the rarest form of fibroid tumour, and occur when a fibroid attaches itself to another organ.

Diagnosis

Diagnosis of uterine fibroids is by physical examination, during which a mass is felt, and by USS.

Treatment

If fibroids are severe enough to cause certain symptoms, surgery is often the required treatment. Symptoms which justify surgery include the following:

- extremely heavy bleeding during the menstrual cycle, which causes anaemia that does not respond to treatment
- pain which has become intolerable, or discomfort caused by the pressure of the fibroids on another organ
- cases where the location of the fibroid is likely to cause further problems.

Surgery for fibroids includes myomectomy and hysterectomy.

Myomectomy is the surgical removal of each individual fibroid without damaging the uterus, thus preserving the ability to conceive. However, fibroids will often grow back, and although it is possible to have a myomectomy repeated, multiple myomectomies can cause other problems, such as the walls of the uterus sticking together due to scarring.

Uterine artery embolisation is a non-surgical procedure that leaves the uterus intact. Polyvinyl particles are inserted into the uterine artery at a point just before the nexus of blood vessels spreads out into the uterine tissue. The particles flow into the vessels and clog them. This prevents the fibroids from receiving the constant blood supply they require, and thus causes them to shrink over time. There is an immediate significant reduction in the symptoms of heavy bleeding and pelvic pain.

As fibroids do grow back, a hysterectomy may be the best option. Removal of the uterus is the only permanent way to effectively relieve most women of fibroids.

Resources

www.fibroids.co.uk
www.fibroidnetworkonline.com

Ovarian cyst

An ovarian cyst is a fluid-filled sac-like structure that develops from one of the ovaries. The majority of ovarian cysts are not tumours, but simple structures termed functional or physiological cysts. These occur as part of the normal physiological functions of the ovary throughout the menstrual cycle. Ovarian cysts are very common and can develop at any age. They are most common in premenopausal women, among whom ovarian cysts occur in 30% of those with regular periods and 50% of those with irregular periods. In addition, ovarian cysts occur in 6% of post-menopausal women. In the latter these are not functional cysts (as there is no ovulation), but may be simple in structure.

During a normal menstrual cycle, small follicles develop on the surface of the ovary, one of which enlarges to 2–3 cm in diameter. At ovulation, the dominant follicle ruptures and releases the egg. The follicle is then transformed into a structure called the corpus luteum, the function of which is to produce the pregnancy hormone progesterone if fertilisation takes place (until the placenta takes over this role). If fertilisation does not occur, the corpus luteum shrivels and disappears.

Functional cysts arise from either the follicle or the corpus luteum. Follicular cysts develop when ovulation does not occur and the follicle continues to grow. Functional cysts can also develop if the corpus luteum persists after ovulation beyond its normal 2-week phase.

Functional cysts may be stimulated by excessive amounts of the female hormones FSH and βHCG. These and other agents may be used to induce ovulation in infertility patients, who thus have an increased risk of developing functional cysts. In contrast, the combined oral contraceptive pill reduces the likelihood of developing functional cysts because it suppresses ovulation.

Symptoms

Most simple ovarian cysts do not produce symptoms unless they have associated complications. Symptoms that may occur include the following:

- lower abdominal pain or discomfort
- fullness or bloating
- pain during sexual intercourse
- urinary frequency or difficulty with bowel movements (because of pressure on adjacent pelvic anatomy)
- irregular periods or spotting.

Ovarian cysts may rupture, twist, bleed or become infected, all of which are likely to cause severe pain and may cause nausea and vomiting. Rupture of a cyst often occurs after exercise, sexual intercourse, trauma or even a pelvic examination. Torsion (twisting) and haemorrhage are more likely to occur in right-sided ovarian cysts.

Diagnosis

- Pelvic/bimanual examination.
- Pelvic USS.

Treatment

If ultrasound examination identifies that the cyst is simple, a 'wait-and-see' plan ('expectant management') may be appropriate, because many simple ovarian cysts resolve spontaneously. The woman should have a repeat ultrasound 6–8 weeks after the simple cyst was first diagnosed. If the cyst has persisted, the patient is usually referred for surgical evaluation, which is most likely to be performed by laparoscopy.

Ovulation pain

Ovulation is the phase of the menstrual cycle that involves the release of an egg from one of the ovaries. About one in five women experience pain and discomfort during ovulation. The duration of the pain ranges from a few minutes to 48 hours. Ovulation pain is also known as mid-cycle pain or mittelschmerz (German for 'middle pain').

Symptoms

The symptoms of ovulation pain can include the following:

- pain in the lower abdomen, just inside the hip bone (the pain typically occurs about 2 weeks before the menstrual period is due). The pain sensation varies from one individual to another. For example, it may feel like uncomfortable pressure, twinges, sharp pains or cramps
- pain that is felt on the right or left side, depending on which ovary is releasing an egg. The pain may switch from one side to the other from one cycle to the next, or it may remain on one side for a few cycles.

The exact cause of ovulation pain is not clear, but the following theories have been suggested.

- *Emerging follicle theory.* Hormones prompt the ovaries to produce follicles. Each follicle contains an immature egg (ovum), but only one follicle usually survives to maturity. It is believed that ovulation pain is caused by the expanding follicle stretching the membrane of the ovary.
- *Ruptured follicle theory.* When the egg is mature, it bursts from the follicle. This may cause slight bleeding. The peritoneum (abdominal lining) could be irritated by the blood or fluids from the ruptured follicle, and this may trigger the pain.

Pelvic/vulval abscess

A pelvic abscess most commonly follows acute appendicitis or gynaecological infections. In women the abscess lies between the uterus and the posterior fornix of the vagina, and the rectum posteriorly. Clinical features include systemic features of toxicity (malaise, nausea, vomiting, pyrexia) and local effects (e.g. diarrhoea, mucous discharge from the rectum, presence of a mass on rectal or vaginal examination). Treatment with antibiotics is successful for early abscesses, otherwise surgical drainage is necessary.

Pelvic congestion

Pelvic congestion is a syndrome that is characterised by symptoms of chronic pelvic pain, congestive dysmenorrhoea, deep dyspareunia and problems related to fluid retention (e.g. swollen fingers, abdominal distension, breast tenderness). There may be excessive cervical secretion which in turn causes vaginal discharge. There may also be reduced libido and failure to achieve orgasm. The pelvic pain is often worse when the patient is walking or standing, and premenstrually. Examination may reveal tenderness, particularly over the ovaries. Vaginal and cervical examination may reveal an apparent blue coloration due to congestion of the pelvic veins. The patient may also have varicose veins of the legs. Investigation for endometriosis and pelvic inflammatory disease should be instigated.

Management options include drug treatment (e.g. medroxyprogesterone for 3 months, which may lead to a symptomatic improvement), bilateral ovarian vein ligation or hysterectomy plus bilateral salpingo-oophorectomy (with postoperative hormone replacement therapy).

Pelvic fistula

In medicine, a *fistula* is an abnormal connection or passageway between organs or vessels that do not normally connect. Fistulas are usually the result of injury or surgery, but can also result from infection or inflammation.

Pelvic inflammatory disease

Pelvic inflammatory disease (PID) is an infection of the upper genital tract. It can affect the uterus, ovaries, Fallopian tubes or other related structures. If left untreated, PID causes scarring and can lead to infertility, tubal pregnancy, chronic pelvic pain and other serious consequences.

PID occurs when disease-causing organisms migrate upward from the urethra and cervix into the upper genital tract. Many different organisms can cause PID, but most cases are associated with gonorrhoea and genital chlamydial infections (two very common STIs).

Symptoms

The major symptoms of PID are as follows:

- lower abdominal pain
- abnormal vaginal discharge.

Other symptoms can include:

- fever
- pain in the right upper abdomen
- pain during intercourse
- irregular menstrual bleeding.

PID can be asymptomatic, particularly when caused by chlamydial infection.

Diagnosis

- Physical examination to determine the nature and location of any pain.
- Fever.
- Abnormal vaginal or cervical discharge.
- Evidence of cervical chlamydial infection or gonorrhoea.

If more information is necessary, the following tests may also be useful:

- USS
- endometrial biopsy
- laparoscopy.

Treatment

Because cultures of specimens from the upper genital tract are difficult to obtain and multiple organisms may be responsible for an episode of PID, especially if it is not the first episode, at least two antibiotics are required (one for bacteria and one for anaerobes) that are effective against a wide range of infectious agents. Patients with a diagnosis of PID should be reviewed to ensure the efficacy of treatment.

Sometimes the symptoms of chronic pain can be improved by surgery.

Consequences of PID

Women with recurrent episodes of PID are more likely than women who have only had a single episode to suffer scarring of the tubes that leads to infertility, tubal pregnancy or chronic pelvic pain. Infertility occurs in approximately 20% of women who have had PID.

However, most women with tubal infertility have never had symptoms of PID. Organisms such as *Chlamydia* can silently invade the Fallopian tubes and cause scarring, which blocks the normal passage of eggs into the uterus.

Another complication of PID is the risk of recurrence of the disease. Up to one-third of women who have had PID will have the disease at least once more. With each episode of reinfection, the risk of infertility is increased.

Resources

www.womenshealthlondon.org.uk/leaflets/pid/pidiag.html
www.medinfo.co.uk/conditions/pid.html
www.netdoctor.co.uk/diseases/facts/pelvicinflammatorydisease.htm

Pelvic organ prolapse

Many women who have given birth may develop a pelvic organ prolapse. During childbirth, the tissues and muscles that hold the pelvic organs in place may become stretched or weakened, and the organs may move from their natural positions to press or bulge into the vagina. For some women, pelvic organ prolapse becomes a painful or uncomfortable problem. However, it is not always a progressive condition, and it may improve over time.

Pelvic organ prolapse is most commonly caused by pregnancy, labour and childbirth. However, it can also be associated with any condition that causes increased pressure in the abdomen, such as obesity, respiratory problems with a chronic cough, constipation, and pelvic organ cancers. Pelvic organ prolapse can also occur after hysterectomy.

Although many women who have pelvic organ prolapse do not have symptoms, the most common and bothersome symptom is bulging or drooping of the uterus into or outside of the vagina. Other symptoms include the following:

- a feeling of pelvic fullness or pressure
- the sensation of something actually falling out of the vagina
- a pulling or stretching in the groin area, or a low backache
- pain during intercourse
- spotting or bleeding from the vagina
- urinary problems, such as incontinence or a frequent or urgent need to urinate, especially at night
- difficulty with bowel movements, such as constipation or needing to support the back of the vagina in order to defecate.

Treatment

Treatment decisions should take into account which organs are affected, the severity of the symptoms, and whether other medical conditions are present. Other important factors are age and sexual activity.

Treatment options fall into two main categories:

- exercises
- use of a removable pessary that is placed inside the vagina to support areas of pelvic organ prolapse.

Resources

www.womenshealthlondon.org.uk/leaflets/prolapse/prolapse.html

Polycystic ovarian syndrome

Polycystic ovarian syndrome (PCOS) is a complex endocrine disorder associated with a long-term lack of ovulation and an excess of androgens. The disorder is characterised by the formation of eight or more follicular cysts of diameter up to 10 mm in the ovaries – a process that is related to the ovary's failure to release an egg. PCOS is one of the commonest causes of infertility.

Symptoms

The common symptoms of PCOS are as follows:

- menstrual irregularity
- acne, excessively oily skin or hairiness (hirsutism) due to excess male-type hormones
- infertility
- weight gain.

Menstrual disturbance

PCOS often comes to light during puberty, due to period problems, which affect around 75% of patients with the condition. Infrequent, irregular or absent periods are all common variations, and many individuals find their periods particularly heavy when they do arrive. The menstrual disturbance is a sign that there is a problem with regular monthly ovulation. Many teenagers use the contraceptive pill to control their periods, as irregular or heavy periods are a common complaint at this time, even in the absence of PCOS. This often leads to a delay in the diagnosis of PCOS, as many women do not present until the pill has been stopped and they find that their periods cease altogether or become irregular.

Androgenic symptoms

Androgens are a group of hormones, such as testosterone, high levels of which occur in men but much lower levels in women. Patients with PCOS often have higher than normal levels of androgens, which may cause excess hairiness, acne and male-pattern hair loss.

Infertility

Given that the menstrual disruption associated with PCOS is due to irregular or absent ovulation, it is not surprising that it is a common cause of infertility. It is not usually absolute, and some women with PCOS will ovulate normally, some will ovulate less frequently and some will not ovulate at all, which means that for some treatment will definitely be necessary.

Obesity

Around 40% of individuals with PCOS are overweight. Obesity itself will initiate the symptoms described above in some women who would not have developed the condition if they had remained of normal weight. Obesity will also worsen the symptoms for those who do have PCOS, and unfortunately the hormone changes associated with PCOS make weight loss more difficult.

Diagnosis

Part of the diagnosis involves observing the symptoms mentioned above.
    Other tests that are used to confirm the diagnosis include the following.

Ultrasound scan

There are multiple small cysts around the edge of the ovaries. These cysts are only a few millimetres in diameter, do not themselves cause problems, and are partially developed eggs that were not released.

Blood tests

A couple of blood tests will assist in making the diagnosis – one to check the level of androgens (such as testosterone), and another to measure the hormones involved in egg development (in PCOS there is a characteristic increase in *luteinising hormone (LH)* levels).

What is the difference between polycystic ovaries (PCO) and polycystic ovarian syndrome (PCOS)?

The term 'polycystic ovaries' describes the ovaries as seen on ultrasound scan. Many women have ovaries that are polycystic, but do not have any of the other symptoms or hormone findings described previously. Overall, around 20% of women in the general population have ovaries with this appearance, and so far research has not identified whether this is one end of a whole spectrum that includes the full polycystic ovary syndrome, or a sign that symptoms are more likely to develop in the future.

Diabetes, insulin and long-term risks

PCOS is closely related to problems with insulin. Insulin is a hormone that is released from the pancreas after a meal, and it allows the organs of the body to take up energy in the form of glucose. In PCOS the cells in the body are resistant to insulin, so the pancreas makes more insulin to try to compensate for this. The excessively high levels of insulin have an effect on the ovary, preventing ovulation and causing a rise in androgen levels.

The long-term risks of PCOS are related to both the insulin problem and the high androgen levels. High levels of insulin are associated with an increased risk of developing type 2 diabetes. The hormone changes described increase the likelihood of developing high blood pressure and high cholesterol levels, both of which can lead to a greater risk of heart disease. Irregular or infrequent periods in the long term lead to an increased risk of cancer of the lining of the uterus. This is partly due to high levels of the hormone oestrogen, which over-stimulates the lining of the uterus. The absence of ovulation, and the resulting progesterone deficiency, also contributes to this risk.

Treatment

Control of irregular periods

Irregular and heavy periods can be due to problems with ovulation. Although it would seem that restarting ovulation would be the best treatment, this is generally reserved for cases where a pregnancy is desired. The drugs that stimulate the ovaries have other side-effects, making their long-term use inappropriate.

Excess weight is a cause of menstrual problems in women with and without PCOS. Extra oestrogen is produced in fat tissues, and this interferes with ovulation and leads to over-stimulation of the lining of the uterus and heavier periods. Weight reduction will improve cycle control and reduce the heaviness of menstrual flow.

Periods may be controlled by the use of the contraceptive pill or a progesterone-like hormone.

Some women have no periods at all, in which case either the contraceptive pill or cyclical progestogens are advisable to avoid the risk of endometrial cancer.

Infertility treatment

PCOS is found in around 70% of women who have ovulation difficulties that lead to infertility. This is more common in women who are overweight, and as a first-line treatment, weight reduction can be very successful in restarting spontaneous ovulation. The amount of weight that needs to be lost is less than most women might expect – loss of around 5% of the current weight is associated with an increased number of ovulatory cycles.

Clomifene

Clomifene citrate is the drug most commonly used to stimulate ovulation. It is taken in the early days of the cycle (usually days 2 to 6) and results in ovulation in around 80% of women overall, and a 6-month successful pregnancy rate of 45–50%.

Ovarian stimulation

If clomifene treatment is unsuccessful, there are two main alternative approaches. The first is to use injectable hormones to stimulate the ovary to produce eggs. This is known as ovarian stimulation, and where there is an additional sperm-related problem, it is combined with insemination of sperm through the cervix around the time of ovulation (intrauterine insemination, or IUI). The hormone treatment must be monitored by blood tests and USS to avoid over-stimulation.

Multiple pregnancy is always a risk with this type of treatment, but especially so for women with PCOS, whose ovaries are particularly sensitive to the hormones. If ovarian stimulation is unsuccessful, many women resort to *in-vitro* fertilisation (IVF), the success rates of which are highly dependent upon individual characteristics such as age, duration of infertility and weight.

Neither IVF nor ovarian stimulation is likely to be successful if a woman is overweight (body mass index greater than 30kg/m^2). For this reason, most hospitals restrict these treatments until the woman's weight is within the normal range.

Laparoscopic ovarian diathermy (LOD) (also known as 'ovarian drilling')

This involves a day-case laparoscopic operation under a short general anaesthetic. The ovaries are identified and several small holes are made in each ovary, either with a fine hot diathermy probe or via a laser. It is not actually known how this procedure works, but it can restore regular ovulation, or make the ovary more sensitive to clomifene.

By 12 months after LOD, the average pregnancy rate is around 60–80%. The highest success rates are obtained in women with a shorter duration of infertility (less than 3 years) and higher levels of luteinising hormone. The advantages of LOD include the fact that it may improve other symptoms of PCOS, such as menstrual disturbance, as well as avoiding the need for stimulatory drugs in order to become pregnant, with their associated increased risk of over-stimulation and multiple pregnancy.

Weight loss

Weight loss will regulate periods, lead to more ovulatory cycles, reduce hairiness, reduce the risk of heart disease and lower insulin levels.

Hirsutism

Hirsutism is usually due to higher than average levels of androgens – the male hormones that are normally present in women at low levels. Initial treatments include bleaching and electrolysis. If these do not produce an acceptable result, drugs may be used to reduce high androgen levels.

The contraceptive pill contains oestrogen, which reduces androgen levels and will improve hirsutism. A formulation is available which includes a specific drug to reduce these further, known as 'Dianette.' One component of Dianette is cyproterone acetate, and this is the next drug to try if hirsutism persists. It is used at a higher dose than that contained in the Dianette pill, but must be combined with adequate contraception, as it can cause fetal abnormality if taken during early pregnancy. Spironolactone is another alternative, but this frequently causes erratic periods, so is often given with a low-dose contraceptive pill.

All hirsutism treatments must be continued for 8–18 months before a response can be expected, due to the slow rate of hair growth. During that time, electrolysis can be performed to remove the unwanted hairs that are already present, and less regrowth can be expected.

Insulin-sensitising drugs – metformin

PCOS can lead to resistance to insulin, as a result of which the body produces excessively high levels of insulin in an attempt to compensate. These higher levels are known to cause abnormal cholesterol and lipid levels, obesity, irregular periods, higher levels of androgens, infertility due to disturbance of ovulation, and an increased likelihood of diabetes. Metformin is a type of drug known as an *insulin-sensitising agent*, which lowers the blood sugar levels, in turn reducing the excessively high insulin levels.

Long-term monitoring

Longer-term risks that have been identified, particularly in women who are overweight, include high blood pressure, high cholesterol levels, and increased risk of diabetes, heart disease and cancer of the lining of the uterus.

Resources

www.soulcysters.com
www.pcosupport.org
www.womens-health.co.uk

Polyps

Cervical polyps

The cervix is a tube-like channel that connects the uterus to the vagina. Cervical polyps are growths that most commonly appear on the cervix at the point where it opens into the vagina. Polyps are usually cherry-red to reddish-purple or greyish-white in colour. They vary in size, and often resemble bulbs on thin stems. Cervical polyps are usually benign, and may occur alone or in groups. Most polyps are small, about 1 to 2 cm long. Because rare types of cancerous conditions can resemble polyps, all polyps should be removed and examined for signs of cancer. The cause of cervical polyps is not well understood, but they are associated with inflammation of the cervix. They may also result from an abnormal response to oestrogen. Cervical polyps are relatively common, especially in women over 20 years of age who have had at least one child. They are rare in girls who have not started to menstruate.

There are two types of cervical polyps.

- *Ectocervical polyps* can develop from the outer surface layer of cells of the cervix. They are more common in post-menopausal women.

- *Endocervical polyps* develop from cervical glands inside the cervical canal. Most cervical polyps are endocervical polyps. They are more common in pre-menopausal women.

Symptoms

Cervical polyps may not cause any symptoms. However, there may be:

- discharge, which can be malodorous if there is an infection
- bleeding between periods
- heavier bleeding during periods
- bleeding after intercourse.

Diagnosis

As most cervical polyps are asymptomatic, they are most often detected during a sexual health screen or cervical smear test. Sometimes a polyp will become detached during sexual intercourse or menstruation. However, most polyps need to be removed so that any symptoms can be treated and the tissue can be evaluated for signs of cancer.

Treatment

Cervical polyps are removed surgically. Polyp forceps are used to grasp the base of the polyp stem and then pluck the polyp with a gentle, twisting motion. Bleeding is usually brief and limited.

Antibiotics may be required if the polyp shows signs of infection. If the polyp is cancerous, treatment will depend on the extent and type of cancer.

Large polyps and polyps with very broad stems usually need to be removed in an operating room using local, regional or general anesthesia. Cervical polyps may grow again from different areas of the cervix, but not usually from the original site. Regular pelvic examination will help to identify and treat polyps before they cause symptoms.

Endometrial polyps

Endometrial polyps are localised overgrowths of the endometrium that project into the uterine cavity. Such polyps may be sessile (broad-based) or pedunculate, and very occasionally include areas of benign or malignant growth. Endometrial polyps are estimated to occur in 10–24% of women undergoing hysterectomy or localised endometrial biopsy. Endometrial polyps are rare among women under 20 years of age. The incidence of these polyps rises steadily with increasing age, peaks in the fifth decade of life, and declines after the menopause.

Symptoms

- Irregular, acyclic uterine bleeding.
- Post-menstrual spotting.

- Prolonged and/or profuse uterine bleeding.
- Post-menopausal bleeding.
- Breakthrough bleeding during hormonal therapy.

Diagnosis

- USS and hysteroscopy.
- Microscopic examination of a specimen obtained after endometrial biopsy or after D&C (dilation and curettage).

Treatment

Treatment is by surgical or hysteroscopic removal.

Useful resources

www.womenshealth.about.com/od/endometrialpolyps
www.fibroids.net/html/polyps.htm

Pyometra

In elderly women with an atrophied cervix and obliterated cervical canal, the development of a uterine infection causes the accumulation of pus that cannot escape. Pyometra can also occur secondary to endometrial or cervical carcinoma. The uterus may perforate. Pyometra accounts for 4 in 10,000 gynaecological admissions.

Vaginismus

Vaginismus occurs when the muscles around the vagina tighten involuntarily, causing the vagina to spasm and possibly causing pain. It is a psychological problem that is manifested in a physical way, and is fairly common. The vaginal muscles go into spasm, usually in response to the vagina or vulva being touched before sexual intercourse. It can also occur if penetration of the vagina by the penis is attempted, or during a gynaecological examination. Vaginismus can cause emotional distress and relationship problems. Women who have vaginismus are able to achieve orgasm during mutual masturbation, foreplay and oral sex. It is only when sexual intercourse is suggested or attempted that the vagina tightens to prevent penetration.

There are many factors that can cause vaginismus. Some women may have had the condition all their adult life and may never have had sexual intercourse because of it. In other cases, vaginismus may be due to other causes, such as the following:

- a physical cause, such as an injury, or inflammation of the vagina, pelvis or bladder
- persistent vaginal dryness or irritation due to spermicides or latex in condoms

- fear or dislike of sex, which may be related to difficult or painful sexual intercourse
- a side-effect of alcohol, medication or drugs
- unpleasant sexual experiences at a young age, or the first sexual experience
- experiencing a past or recent trauma to the genital area or an incident linked to sexuality
- sexual abuse, assault or rape
- a very strict upbringing in which sex was never discussed, or unhelpful comments leading to feelings of guilt and shame
- religious or cultural taboos
- fear of getting pregnant
- relationship problems
- after a vaginal infection
- the after-effects of childbirth, including tiredness and depression
- inadequate sex education, or being told that sex is painful or that sexual desire is wrong, resulting in fear and anxiety about sex.

Even if the original physical cause has disappeared, vaginismus can still continue to occur.

Diagnosis

The diagnosis is based on the woman's medical history, the symptoms and a physical examination, if possible.

Treatment

Any physical disorders that may be causing or contributing to vaginismus will need to be treated – for example, an injury or infection. If the cause of the condition is psychological, counselling for the woman and her partner (if she is in a relationship) will be necessary. If the cause is less obvious, it may be a case of taking time to see whether the problem resolves itself with self-help techniques.

Useful resources

www.vaginismus.com

Vulval intra-epithelial neoplasia

Vulval intra-epithelial neoplasia (VIN) is the pre-invasive phase of carcinoma of the vulva. It affects 20–30 per 100,000 women, and approximately 40% of cases occur in women under 41 years of age. Proposed aetiological factors include human papilloma virus and immunosuppression. Clinical features include pruritus vulvae and abnormal skin lesions of the vulva. A skin biopsy is required. Management includes local excision and careful monitoring, as approximately 6% of lesions become malignant. Topical steroids may have a role in symptomatic treatment. If VIN is diagnosed, there is a greater than 10% risk of neoplasia elsewhere, generally cervical, and examination of the cervix and breasts should be undertaken.

Vulval tuberculosis

Vulval tuberculosis occurs in conjunction with TB of the upper genital tract. On examination there may be an ulcer with blue, undetermined edges. For individuals who come from areas where pulmonary TB is prevalent, genitourinary TB (GUTB) is a common site of extrapulmonary TB (accounting for 15–20% of extrapulmonary cases).

When it does occur, the disease can involve the kidney, ureter, bladder or genital organs. Clinical features usually develop 10–15 years after the primary infection. Only about 25% of patients with GUTB have a known history of tuberculosis. The true incidence and prevalence of GUTB are difficult to estimate, because a large number of patients remain asymptomatic.

Useful resources

www.sunmed.org/pelvictb.html

Hormonal conditions

- **Adrenal hyperplasia**

- **Craniopharyngioma**

- **Early menopause**

- **Hyperprolactinoma**

- **Menopause**

- **Pituitary cancer**

- **Pituitary disorders (hyperpituitarism and hypopituitarism)**

- **Premenstrual dysphoric disorder**

- **Premenstrual syndrome (PMS)**

- **Thyroid disorders (hyperthyroidism, hypothyroidism and hyper-parathyroidism)**

Adrenal hyperplasia

Congenital adrenal hyperplasia (CAH) is a metabolic disorder related to enzymatic defects in the biosynthesis of cortical steroids. Typically the defects are inherited in an autosomal recessive manner.

The adrenal gland sits above each kidney, one on each side of the body. It is made up of two parts:

- the *adrenal medulla*, which makes adrenaline and the outer part of the adrenal gland
- the *adrenal cortex*, which makes three main steroid hormones that are secreted into the bloodstream and are necessary for normal health. It is the adrenal cortex and its hormones which are involved in CAH.

The three main steroid hormones involved in CAH are cortisol, aldosterone and androgens.

- *Cortisol* controls how the body copes with emotional and physical stress, including infection and injury. It also helps to control blood sugar levels, raising the levels if they become too low.

- *Aldosterone* helps to regulate the salt levels in the body. It causes the kidneys to conserve salt if there is too little salt in the diet, or if large amounts of salt are lost due to excessive sweating. Conversely, if a large amount of salt is consumed in the diet, the adrenal cortex reduces the amount of aldosterone secreted, allowing the excess salt to be excreted in the urine.
- *Androgens* are a group of male hormones, one of which is testosterone. Testosterone is produced by the adrenal cortex in both males and females, and it controls the formation of pubic hair at the onset of puberty. Testosterone is also produced by the testis, and in small amounts by the ovary.

There are five main enzymes in the adrenal gland which convert cholesterol into cortisol. If any of these enzymes are missing or defective, insufficient cortisol is produced for the needs of the body. The body, recognising the low levels of cortisol, will try to stimulate the adrenal cortex to make more cortisol by means of a stimulating hormone called adrenocorticotropic hormone (ACTH), which is produced by the pituitary gland. The constant unsuccessful stimulation causes the cortex to increase in thickness and become *hyperplastic*.

Different types of CAH

There are many different grades of severity of CAH depending on the degree of impairment of production of cortisol and aldosterone. In the most severe type of CAH, aldosterone is completely lacking and loss of salt from the body is the most prominent problem – *salt-losing CAH* accounts for 80% of children with CAH. The loss of salt in the urine is uncontrolled and can cause acute dehydration, very low blood pressure and vomiting. The levels of salt and glucose in the blood fall, and the level of potassium rises. This is known as an *adrenal crisis*, and requires very urgent treatment as it is a potentially life-threatening condition.

With less severe CAH, also known as *non-salt-losing CAH*, the salt balance is normal. However, in stressful situations some people with non-salt-losing CAH may become salt losers and require extra treatment. Girls born with non-salt-losing CAH are usually healthy, but are often born with an enlarged clitoris and the labia may be partially fused because of the excess testosterone. In general, this is less severe than that seen in salt-losing cases. In boys, non-salt-losing CAH produces no detectable signs at birth, and the diagnosis is made when the penis enlarges at a very early age along with early pubic hair and rapid growth in height resulting from high levels of testosterone. These changes may not occur until 4 or 5 years of age.

The mildest form of CAH, known as *late-onset CAH*, can affect women of any age. Symptoms of unwanted hair growth or irregular periods can start at any time after puberty. Often treatment with steroids is not necessary in women with late-onset CAH. Instead, giving oestrogen – for example, as the combined oral contraceptive – can regulate testosterone production by the ovary. Treatment of late-onset CAH is usually the same as that for PCOS because the two conditions are so similar. In men, late-onset CAH usually goes unrecognised, although it may result in a low sperm count.

Treatment

- Treatment aims to provide lifelong replacement hydrocortisone and a salt-retaining steroid. This will inhibit ACTH secretion and so reduce adrenal androgen production.
- Surgical correction of the masculinised female genitalia is performed in the first year of life.
- A salt-losing crisis requires urgent intravenous saline, glucose and hydrocortisone.

Useful resources

www.congenitaladrenalhyperplasia.org
www.cah.org.uk

Craniopharyngioma

A craniopharyngioma is a brain tumour that can occur at any age, but which is most commonly found during childhood or adolescence. These tumours are not usually detected until they impinge upon important structures around them. As a result, they are often quite large when they are eventually detected, ranging from an average of about 2 cm in diameter to more than 6 cm. They are almost always benign.

Symptoms

Symptoms produced by the tumour vary depending on the location. If the tumour compresses the pituitary stalk or involves the pituitary gland itself, it can cause pituitary hormone deficiency. If it involves the optic tracts, chiasm or nerves, visual problems can result. Involvement of the hypothalamus (which is located at the base of the brain) may result in obesity, increased drowsiness, temperature regulation abnormalities or diabetes insipidus. Common symptoms include personality changes, headache, confusion and vomiting.

Diagnosis

- Medical history and examination.
- CT and MRI scan.
- Hormone levels in relation to possibly implicated structures.

Treatment

The initial treatment most commonly involves surgery. The goal of surgery is to remove the entire tumour, while improving or preserving the pituitary, visual and brain function. There are a couple of different surgical options, including surgery that involves access through the nose (trans-sphenoidal surgery), or a craniotomy (in which an opening is made in the skull to allow access to the tumour).

If the tumour cannot be completely removed, radiation treatment is used to increase the likelihood of survival.

Early menopause

Early menopause and premature menopause are terms that are often used interchangeably, and they are frequently used as umbrella terms to cover many different situations and conditions, ranging from premature ovarian failure to menopause caused by surgery, chemotherapy or radiation treatment.

Early menopause refers to menopause (i.e. total cessation of periods for 12 months) that occurs before the age of 45 years.

Premature menopause refers to menopause that occurs before the age of 40 years. If premature menopause occurs naturally (i.e. menopause is not due to surgery, radiation treatment or chemotherapy), it is more commonly referred to as *premature ovarian failure*.

Causes of premature ovarian failure

Autoimmune disorder

In autoimmune disorder, the body's immune system attacks itself. There may be production of antibodies to ovarian tissue, endometrium, or one or more of the hormones that regulate ovulation. These antibodies attack the reproductive system, and may interfere with and eventually destroy ovarian function. If there is a personal or family history of autoimmune disorders (such as thyroid disease, diabetes or rheumatoid arthritis), this may be the cause of early menopause.

Chromosomal irregularity

Some cases of hereditary premature menopause are caused by defects on an X chromosome. Fragile X syndrome interferes with the production of eggs, and the production of a smaller number of eggs by the ovaries leads to an earlier menopause, generally 6 to 8 years before that in other women. Another related form of genetically caused premature menopause is Turner's syndrome, where there is no second X chromosome, or a part of the chromosome is missing. Since two X chromosomes are required for the ovaries to develop properly, a missing or faulty X chromosome leads to impairment of ovarian development. Often women with Turner's syndrome never have periods at all, because their ovaries never develop properly and do not produce ovarian oestrogen. In some women, premature menopause occurs because they have three X chromosomes, which also interferes with ovarian development.

Surgical causes of early menopause

Oophorectomy and total hysterectomy

This is one of the commonest causes of early menopause. Premature menopause is experienced after removal of both the ovaries (a bilateral oophorectomy) or removal of the uterus, both Fallopian tubes and both ovaries (a total hysterectomy). Because both ovaries are removed, oestrogen and progesterone levels fall dramatically, leading immediately to menopause. Because of this sudden drop in levels, the symptoms may be more intense than those experienced by women who go into premature menopause spontaneously.

Ovarian damage due to other surgical procedures

So long as there is one ovary, hormones are usually still produced and premature menopause should not occur. However, in some cases after a hysterectomy in which one or both ovaries are left intact, one or both of them may fail, either immediately after surgery or up to a few years later. This may also happen when the ovary or ovaries are damaged or otherwise affected by procedures such as cyst removal, or when the surgery damages blood vessels and thus interferes with blood flow to the ovaries. In such cases the follicles on the remaining ovary or ovaries slowly die out, resulting in menopause. Similarly, some women experience premature menopause after tubal ligation. Again this is a result of the surgery interfering with blood flow to the ovaries, which eventually leads to ovarian failure.

Causes of chemical early menopause

Radiation therapy and/or chemotherapy

With the rise in cancer treatments there has been an increase in premature menopause due to these treatments. Unfortunately, the significant doses of radiation or chemotherapy used to kill cancer cells can also damage the ovaries, resulting in premature menopause. In some cases, especially if there has been low-dose and/or short-term treatment, temporary menopause due to chemotherapy or radiation therapy may be experienced. Even when the woman's periods return, she may be infertile.

Tamoxifen

Tamoxifen used to be prescribed for breast cancer, and premature menopause can be a side-effect of this drug. Recently, doctors have begun to prescribe tamoxifen as a preventive treatment for women at high risk for breast cancer, as it reduces breast cancer rates by about 45%. Although there are many positive aspects of treatment with this drug, premature menopause is a possibility. This is because tamoxifen takes the place that oestrogen would occupy, thus acting as an oestrogen-blocker. Since the body is not receiving the normal amount of oestrogen, low oestrogen levels signal the body to produce more FSH, and the body may ultimately react by entering the menopause prematurely. Often this is only a temporary effect and normal ovarian function eventually returns.

Other causes

- Family history.
- Viral infections. If a woman contracts a viral infection while she is pregnant, the infection can affect the ovarian development of the fetus, leading to a

lower number of eggs. Therefore in adulthood that individual can run out of eggs more quickly, resulting in premature menopause. Some studies suggest that a small number of women may experience premature menopause if they have had mumps and the infection spread to their ovaries.

Useful resources

www.earlymenopause.com

Hyperprolactinoma

A prolactinoma is a prolactin-producing tumour of the pituitary gland. It is a benign tumour. Prolactinomas only grow very slowly, and many do not seem to grow at all. They vary in size, but the vast majority are less than 10 mm in diameter. These are called microprolactinomas. The rarer larger tumours are called macroprolactinomas. The symptoms produced by a prolactinoma depend on the sex of the patient and the size of the tumour, and include the following:

- loss of periods, as excessive prolactin interferes with the pituitary gland's production of FSH and LH, which control the menstrual cycle
- reduced interest in sex, and vaginal dryness and discomfort during intercourse
- infertility due to impaired release of eggs by the ovaries
- excess production of breast milk (galactorrhoea), which may leak spontaneously. This is simply due to the biological action of prolactin, and is *not* a sign of breast disease.

Diagnosis

- Blood tests – prolactin levels, TFTs.
- CT or MRI scan.

Treatment

Drug treatment is used to reduce prolactin secretion by the prolactinoma. This treatment reverses the symptoms as prolactin secretion decreases and the tumour shrinks. If drug treatment is not well tolerated, surgery is occasionally recommended.

Useful resources

www.pituitary.org.uk/resources/prolactinoma.htm

Menopause

The menopause literally means the last menstrual period. It indicates primary ovarian failure, and on average it occurs at 51 years of age in women in the UK.

Physiologically, it is characterised by increased production of FSH and LH as negative feedback from serum oestrogen diminishes.

The menopause occurs when the supply of responsive oocytes is exhausted. Ovarian function does not cease instantaneously. Symptoms of impending failure may be apparent several months or years before the last menstrual period. This is known as the perimenopause or climacteric, and it is what most laypeople refer to as the menopause. Similarly, symptoms may persist for several years afterwards.

The perimenopause is characterised by an increased proportion of anovulatory cycles. As a result, progesterone production is decreased, secretory endometrial changes are less marked, and menses become irregular.

A woman is regarded as post-menopausal from 1 year after her final menstrual period.

After the menopause, oestrogen production falls as the major source of oestradiol – the granulosa cells of the developing follicle is lost. Thus the negative feedback on pituitary production of FSH and LH by oestrogen is reduced. Serum levels of FSH and LH rise, and values greater than 40 IU/l indicate post-menopausal status.

Symptoms

- Hot flushes.
- Sleep problems.
- Depression and mood swings.
- Vaginal problems, including vaginal dryness and irritation that can cause pain during intercourse and gynaecological examinations, as well as frequent vaginal infections.
- Urinary problems, including burning or pain when urinating, or stress incontinence (the weakening of tissues in the urinary tract, which causes urine to leak when one is sneezing, coughing or laughing).
- Memory loss.
- Changes in sex drive and sexual response.
- Weight gain.
- Hair loss.
- 'Spotting' and abnormal bleeding (this is usually normal, but should be reported to a doctor).

Treatment

Hormone replacement therapy (HRT) is the mainstay of treatment in this condition.

However, other therapies are effective in certain situations, either as alternatives or as a supplement to HRT. These include the following:

- clonidine – for relief of hot flushes
- beta-blockers – for relief of palpitations and tachycardia
- antidepressants, sedatives and hypnotics – for relief of non-vasomotor symptoms
- calcium, calcitonins, vitamin D supplements and exercise – for prevention of osteoporosis

- psychological support – the marked placebo effect in several studies points to the value of psychological support and a sympathetic ear. The menopause frequently coincides with other stresses – such as children leaving home – which may exacerbate the biological changes associated with this time of life.

Useful resources

www.menopausematters.co.uk
www.menopause-online.com

Pituitary cancer

The pituitary gland controls several hormone glands, including the thyroid, adrenal and reproductive glands. It is usually about the size of a pea, and is situated in a bony hollow beneath the base of the brain, behind the bridge of the nose.

The pituitary gland produces a number of hormones, including prolactin, FSH and LH. Prolactin is sometimes known as the 'milk hormone' because it stimulates milk production after childbirth. FSH and LH control sex and reproduction. In women they cause release of the sex hormone oestrogen and stimulate the ovaries to produce eggs. These hormones are essential for a normal menstrual cycle.

A pituitary tumour can be either benign or malignant. Although a benign tumour may continue to grow, the cells do not spread from the original site. In a malignant tumour, the cells can invade and destroy the surrounding tissue and may spread to other parts of the brain.

Pituitary tumours are either secreting (hormone-producing) or non-secreting (non-hormone-producing) tumours. Secreting tumours can release excess amounts of any of the pituitary hormones, and are named after the hormone that is being over-produced (e.g. prolactin-secreting tumour).

Pituitary disorders

Hyperpituitarism

This condition is characterised by excessive activity of the pituitary gland, especially overactivity of the anterior lobe (which leads to excess secretion of growth hormone). Although a certain amount of growth hormone is needed by the body for normal regulatory functions, too much results in the abnormal growth of hands, feet and internal organs (acromegaly). Hyperpituitarism is usually caused by a tumour.

Symptoms

Symptoms can include the following:

- headache
- visual field loss or double vision
- excessive sweating
- hoarseness
- milk secretion from the breast

- sleep apnoea
- carpal tunnel syndrome
- joint pain and limitation of motion
- muscle weakness
- numbness or tingling of the skin.

Diagnosis

- History of symptoms.
- Computed tomography (CT or CAT) scan.
- Magnetic resonance imaging (MRI).
- Blood tests to measure hormone levels.

Treatment

Treatment has the following aims:

- to reduce the concentration of growth hormone (GH) and insulin-like growth factor 1 (IGF-1) to a normal level
- to relieve pressure from the pituitary tumour on the optic nerves and surrounding areas of the brain
- to preserve normal pituitary function
- to reverse or improve the symptoms of acromegaly.

Treatment options recommended by the Expert Consensus Guideline for acromegaly include the following:

- surgery to remove the tumour
- drug therapy
- radiation therapy of the pituitary gland.

Hypopituitarism

Hypopituitarism, characterised by an underactive pituitary gland, is a condition that affects the anterior lobe of the pituitary gland, usually resulting in a partial or complete loss of functioning of that lobe.

Symptoms

Symptoms vary depending on which hormones are no longer being produced in sufficient amounts by the pituitary gland. The following are common symptoms associated with reduced production of specific hormones:

- insufficient *gonadotropin* production (luteinising hormone and follicle-stimulating hormone) – in premenopausal women, this leads to absence of menstrual cycles, infertility, vaginal dryness and loss of some female characteristics
- insufficient *growth hormone* production – this does not usually produce any symptoms in adults. In children, this deficiency can lead to stunted growth and dwarfism

- insufficient *thyroid-stimulating hormone* production – this usually leads to an underactive thyroid and may cause confusion, cold intolerance, weight gain, constipation and dry skin
- insufficient *corticotropin* production – this rare deficiency leads to an underactive adrenal gland, resulting in low blood pressure, a low blood sugar level, fatigue and a low stress tolerance
- insufficient *prolactin* production – this rare deficiency may cause an inability to produce breast milk after childbirth in some women.

Causes of hypopituitarism

Causes of hypopituitarism can affect the pituitary gland directly, or may influence it indirectly via the hypothalamus, which in turn affects the pituitary gland.

Causes of primary hypopituitarism (directly affecting the pituitary gland) include the following:

- pituitary tumours
- inadequate blood supply to the pituitary gland
- infections and/or inflammatory diseases
- radiation therapy
- surgical removal of pituitary tissue
- autoimmune disease.

Causes of secondary hypopituitarism (affecting the hypothalamus) include the following:

- tumours of the hypothalamus
- inflammatory disease
- head injuries
- surgical damage to the pituitary gland and/or the blood vessels or nerves leading to it.

Diagnosis

- History of symptoms.
- Computed tomography (CT or CAT) scan.
- Magnetic resonance imaging (MRI).
- Blood tests to measure hormone levels.

Treatment

Treatment of hypopituitarism depends on its cause. The goal of treatment is to restore the pituitary gland to normal function, so that it produces normal levels of hormones. Treatment may include hormone replacement therapy, surgical removal of the tumour and/or radiation therapy.

Premenstrual dysphoric disorder

Premenstrual dysphoric disorder (PMDD) is a diagnosis used to indicate serious premenstrual distress with an associated deterioration in functioning. PMDD is characterised by depressed or labile mood, anxiety, irritability, anger and other symptoms occurring exclusively during the 2 weeks preceding menses. The symptoms must be severe enough to interfere with occupational and social functioning, as opposed to the more common premenstrual syndrome (PMS). PMDD is an extremely distressing and disabling condition that requires treatment.

The treatment of PMDD includes both non-pharmacological and pharmacological approaches. Non-pharmacological treatment includes aerobic exercise, consumption of complex carbohydrates and frequent meals, relaxation training, light therapy, sleep deprivation and cognitive behavioural approaches. Drug treatment may include antidepressants and the combined oral contraceptive pill.

Useful resources

http://pmdd.factsforhealth.org
www.womensmentalhealth.org/resources/ForPatients/pdd.html

Premenstrual syndrome (PMS)

In this condition, certain symptoms occur each month before a period. PMS is sometimes called premenstrual tension (PMT), but increased tension may not be the only symptom.

Symptoms

- Psychological (mental) symptoms include tension, irritability, tiredness, feelings of aggression or anger, low mood, anxiety and feeling emotional. There may be a change in sleep pattern, sexual feelings and appetite. Relationships may become strained because of these symptoms.
- Physical symptoms include breast swelling and/or pain, abdominal bloating, swelling of the hands or feet, weight gain and an increase in the frequency of headaches. People with epilepsy, asthma, migraine or cold sores may find that these conditions become worse before a period.

The cause of PMS is not known. Ovulation appears to trigger symptoms. It is thought that women with PMS are more sensitive to the normal level of progesterone. One effect of over-sensitivity to progesterone seems to be a reduction in the level of a brain chemical (neurotransmitter) called serotonin. This may lead to the symptoms of PMS, and it explains why drugs that increase the serotonin level are effective in women with PMS.

Treatment

- *Exercise.* Some women who exercise regularly report that they have fewer problems with PMS.
- *Food and drink.* Some authors claim that various diets, minerals and supplements help to ease the symptoms of PMS. However, there is little scientific evidence that food, or particular types of food, makes any difference. Some women find that alcohol makes their symptoms worse.

Popular 'over-the-counter' treatments

Vitamin B_6 (pyridoxine) has been used for several years. This vitamin is part of a normal diet, but higher levels are thought to help to relieve the symptoms of PMS. There is only limited evidence that vitamin B_6 is effective, but it is worth a try. It can be taken either 2 weeks before a woman's period, or every day.

Agnus castus fruit extract works well in many cases. In one research study, one tablet of agnus castus extract was taken by women with PMS every day for three menstrual cycles. Over half of the women reported a 50% or greater improvement in their symptoms. It is not clear how agnus castus works, but it contains substances that may affect certain brain chemicals (neurotransmitters).

Other treatments

Selective serotonin reuptake inhibitor (SSRI) medication

SSRIs are commonly prescribed to treat more severe PMS. These medicines were first developed to treat depression. However, they have also been found to ease the symptoms of PMS. They work by increasing the level of serotonin in the brain.

Prevention of ovulation

Prevention of ovulation (e.g. by using the combined oral contraceptive pill) usually prevents the symptoms of PMS. This is because ovulation, and the release of progesterone into the bloodstream after ovulation, seems to trigger the symptoms.

Other treatments

Some women only experience one or two physical symptoms. The following treatments may improve a specific physical symptom, but are unlikely to relieve psychological symptoms (unless the physical symptom is causing or aggravating the irritability, anxiety, etc.).

- Diuretics, in particular spironolactone, can help to reduce fluid retention and bloating.
- Anti-inflammatory painkillers may help if painful symptoms develop.
- Evening primrose oil may ease breast discomfort.

Useful resources

www.pms.org.uk

Thyroid disorders (hyperthyroidism, hypothyroidism and hyperparathyroidism)

The thyroid gland is located in the front of the neck, below the larynx (voice box). This gland is about 3 cm in diameter, and consists of two lobes, one on each side of the windpipe, connected by tissue called the isthmus.

The thyroid tissue is composed of two types of cells – follicular cells and parafollicular cells. Most of the thyroid tissue consists of follicular cells, which secrete iodine-containing hormones called thyroxine (T_4) and tri-iodothyronine (T_3). The parafollicular cells secrete the hormone calcitonin. The thyroid requires iodine in order to produce these hormones.

The thyroid gland plays an important role in regulating the body's metabolism and calcium balance. The T_4 and T_3 hormones stimulate every tissue in the body to produce proteins and increase the amount of oxygen used by cells. The harder the cells work, the harder the organs work. Calcitonin works together with the parathyroid hormone to regulate calcium levels in the body.

The levels of hormones secreted by the thyroid are controlled by the pituitary gland's thyroid-stimulating hormone, which is in turn controlled by the hypothalamus.

Hyperthyroidism (thyrotoxicosis, Grave's disease)

This condition is characterised by overactivity of the thyroid gland, resulting in too much thyroid hormone in the bloodstream. The oversecretion of thyroid hormones leads to overactivity of the body's metabolism.

Symptoms

- These include the following:
- nervousness
- irritability
- increased perspiration
- thinning of the skin
- fine, brittle hair
- weak muscles, especially in the upper arms and thighs
- shaky hands
- fast heartbeat
- high blood pressure
- increased bowel movements
- weight loss
- difficulty in sleeping
- sensitivity of the eyes to light
- staring
- confusion
- irregular menstrual cycle.

Diagnosis

- Measurement of thyroid hormone levels in the bloodstream.
- Thyroid scan, which uses a radioactive substance to create an image of the thyroid as it is functioning.

Treatment

- Antithyroid drugs that help to lower the level of thyroid hormones in the blood.
- Radioactive iodine, in the form of a pill or liquid, which damages thyroid cells so that the production of thyroid hormones is slowed down.

- Surgery to remove part of the thyroid (the overactive nodule).
- Use of beta-blocking agents, which block the action of thyroid hormone on the body.

Hypothyroidism

This condition is characterised by an underactive thyroid. Hypothyroidism is the most common thyroid disorder. Severe hypothyroidism can lead to a condition called myxoedema, characterised by dry, thickened skin and coarse facial features.

The most common cause of hypothyroidism is an autoimmune reaction, in which the body produces antibodies against the thyroid gland. Other causes include treatment of hyperthyroidism, such as radioactive iodine treatment or surgery.

Symptoms

Symptoms of hypothyroidism are usually very subtle and gradual, and may be mistaken for symptoms of depression. They can include the following:

- dull facial expressions
- hoarse voice
- slow speech
- droopy eyelids
- puffy and swollen face
- weight gain
- constipation
- sparse, coarse and dry hair
- coarse, dry and thickened skin
- carpal tunnel syndrome (hand tingling or pain)
- slow pulse
- muscle cramps
- orange-coloured soles and palms
- thinning or falling out of sides of eyebrows
- confusion
- increased menstrual flow in women.

Diagnosis

- A complete medical history and examination.
- Blood tests to measure levels of thyroid hormones and the thyroid-stimulating hormones produced by the pituitary gland.

Treatment

Treatment may include prescription of thyroid hormones to replace the deficient hormones. The dosage of thyroid hormone may need to be increased over the years.

Hyperparathyroidism

The parathyroid glands

The parathyroid glands are two small oval-shaped glands located adjacent to the two thyroid gland lobes in the neck. They produce parathyroid hormone, which plays a role in the regulation of calcium levels in the blood. The maintenance of precise calcium levels in the human body is important, as small deviations from normal can cause muscle and nerve impairment.

Parathyroid hormone stimulates the following functions:

- release of calcium from bone tissue into the bloodstream
- absorption of food by the intestines
- conservation of calcium by the kidneys.

Hyperparathyroidism is caused by overactive parathyroid glands that produce too much parathyroid hormone, which in turn leads to increased levels of calcium in the bloodstream. The excess calcium released from bone tissue leads to osteoporosis and osteomalacia (both of which are bone-weakening diseases). Hyperparathyroidism can also cause kidney stones, due to the high levels of calcium excreted into the urine by the kidneys.

Causes of hyperparathyroidism include benign tumours on the parathyroid glands and enlargement of the parathyroid glands.

Symptoms

Symptoms may include the following:

- aches and pains
- depression
- abdominal pain
- nausea
- vomiting
- fatigue
- excessive urination
- confusion
- muscle weakness.

Diagnosis

- A complete medical history and examination.
- Bone X-rays.
- Laboratory tests to measure calcium and parathyroid hormone levels.

Treatment

Treatment may include removal of parathyroid tissue.

Useful resources

www.thyroid.org
http://thyroid.about.com

Breast conditions

- **Breast cancer**

- **Ectasia**

- **Ectopic prolactin synthesis**

- **Fibroadenoma**

- **Fibrocystic breast disease**

- **Galactocele**

- **Granulomatous lobular mastitis**

- **Hyperprolactinaemia**

- **Intraductal papilloma**

- **Lax cyst**

- **Lipoma**

- **Mastitis**

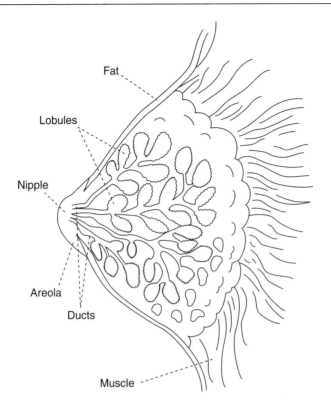

Figure 4 Cross-section through the breast.

Breast cancer

There are several forms of breast cancer:

- ductal carcinoma *in situ*
- lobular carcinoma *in situ*
- phyllodes tumour
- inflammatory breast cancer
- Paget's disease of the breast
- invasive lobular breast cancer
- secondary breast cancer.

Ductal carcinoma in situ

Ductal carcinoma *in situ* (DCIS) is an early form of breast cancer, sometimes described as a pre-cancerous, intraductal or non-invasive cancer. The cancer cells are confined to the milk ducts and have not developed the ability to spread through the breast or outside it. There are a number of different types of DCIS. Based on the appearance of the cells under the microscope, they are graded as high-, intermediate- or low-grade DCIS. If DCIS is left untreated, the cells may eventually spread from the ducts into the surrounding breast tissue and become an invasive cancer.

Symptoms

- Asymptomatic.
- A lump.
- Discharge from the nipple.
- A type of nipple rash known as Paget's disease of the breast.

Diagnosis

As DCIS does not usually have any symptoms, most cases are diagnosed from a mammogram. The latter often shows a cluster of small white dots of calcium, known as microcalcifications. Not all microcalcifications turn out to be DCIS. If there is any doubt, a core biopsy is taken. Symptoms such as a lump or nipple discharge will require a range of tests which may include a mammogram and fine-needle aspiration (FNA).

Treatment

Currently there is no one approach that is suitable for all women, and the treatment offered will depend on factors such as the extent and grade of DCIS.

Surgery
- Mastectomy with or without breast reconstruction.
- Wide local excision.

It is unlikely that the lymph nodes in the axilla will need to be removed for DCIS.

Additional treatments
To reduce the risk of DCIS recurring or invasive cancer developing, other treatments may be given alongside surgery, which include radiotherapy and hormone therapy.

Lobular carcinoma in situ

Breast tissue is composed of ducts and lobules which are supported by fat and connective tissue. Milk is produced and stored within the lobules and carried through to the nipple via the ducts during breastfeeding. In lobular carcinoma *in situ* (LCIS) there are cell changes within the lobules at the end of the ducts. LCIS has been linked to a slightly increased risk of developing breast cancer in the future.

Diagnosis

LCIS is usually found by chance at the breast clinic when the tissue from a biopsy or breast surgery is examined under the microscope in the laboratory.

Treatment

It is unlikely that treatment will be needed, as most women who are diagnosed with LCIS do not develop breast cancer. Regular check-ups are recommended.

A form of hormone therapy may be suggested to try to reduce the likelihood of breast cancer developing.

Phyllodes tumour

Phyllodes tumours are a rare type of breast lump that can affect a woman at any time in her life, although they are most commonly found in premenopausal women between the ages of 40 and 50 years.

Phyllodes tumours are classified into three groups:

- benign (most common)
- borderline malignant
- malignant.

Rarely, a benign phyllodes tumour can recur after it has been removed, and may develop into a borderline malignant or malignant form, although this is very unusual.

Diagnosis

This involves triple assessment:

1 breast examination
2 mammogram or ultrasound scan
3 FNA.

Treatment

Phyllodes tumours are treated by surgery. The surgeon will remove the tumour and an area of healthy tissue around it to reduce the risk of the tumour recurring. A mastectomy may be suggested, depending on the location of the tumour in the breast and how much tissue is affected.

Inflammatory breast cancer

Inflammatory breast cancer is so called because the overlying skin of the breast has a reddened appearance. In patients with inflammatory breast cancer, the reddened appearance is caused by breast cancer cells blocking tiny channels in the breast tissue known as lymph channels. The latter are part of the lymphatic system that is involved in the body's defence against infections. Inflammatory breast cancer is a rare type of breast cancer.

Signs and symptoms

The symptoms of inflammatory breast cancer can appear over a short space of time, and may include the following:

- warmth, redness or swelling of the breast, which may feel sore
- the appearance of ridges on the skin

- the breast may appear pitted like the skin of an orange
- a lump
- pain in the breast or nipple
- a nipple discharge
- the nipple may be inverted.

Diagnosis

Inflammatory breast cancer can be difficult to diagnose because the symptoms may be similar to those of non-cancerous conditions such as mastitis.

A mammogram and ultrasound scan can aid diagnosis, and a confirmatory biopsy is usually performed.

Treatment

Inflammatory breast cancer can grow more quickly than other types of breast cancer, so there is a stronger possibility that cancer cells may spread to other parts of the body. For this reason, treatment is usually started straight away. Treatment usually involves both systemic treatment and local treatment.

A combination of the following treatments may be used:

- chemotherapy
- surgery
- radiotherapy
- hormone therapy.

Paget's disease of the breast

Paget's disease of the nipple is a presentation of breast cancer that is associated with DCIS or invasive carcinoma in the underlying breast. It typically presents as a unilateral red bleeding eczematous lesion of the nipple which is eventually eroded. About 40% of cases present with a palpable lump – a relatively late stage. Rarely, Paget's disease may affect other apocrine gland-bearing areas, such as the vulva.

Management is focused on detection and treatment of any associated malignancy. Total mastectomy with axillary dissection may be preferable in older patients, as it is rapid and reliable. For women who wish to avoid mastectomy, radiotherapy alone or after cone excision of the nipple, areola and underlying ducts may be offered.

Paget's disease with associated intraductal carcinoma only and no palpable lump has an excellent prognosis, with a cure rate approaching 100%.

Invasive lobular breast cancer

Invasive lobular breast cancer is uncommon, and is generally no more serious than other types of breast cancer. However, it is sometimes found in both breasts at the same time, and there is also a slightly higher risk of it occurring in the opposite breast at a later date.

Symptoms

Invasive lobular cancer is more likely to be manifested as a thickening of the breast tissue rather than a definite hard lump. Because the symptoms can be vague, these cancers may sometimes grow to a larger size than other breast cancers before they are detected.

Diagnosis

- Mammogram.
- Ultrasound scan.
- FNA.
- Needle core biopsy.

Treatment

Surgery
- Mastectomy.
- Wide local excision.

It is important to determine whether the cancer has spread to the lymph nodes in the axilla. Some or all of the lymph nodes may be taken. This helps to determine whether other treatment such as chemotherapy will be necessary.

Additional treatment
- Chemotherapy.
- Radiotherapy – this is usually offered after a wide local excision.
- Hormone therapy – the hormone therapy drug tamoxifen may be offered if the tumour is oestrogen receptor positive, which means that it depends on the hormone oestrogen for growth. Most invasive lobular cancers are oestrogen receptor positive.

Secondary breast cancer

Secondary breast cancer occurs when cancer cells break away from the breast and travel through the bloodstream or lymphatic system to other parts of the body. causing further symptoms according to the area in which they have settled.

Useful resources

www.breastcancercare.org.uk

Ectasia

Duct ectasia affects women who are reaching the menopause. The ducts behind the nipple become dilated, which is normal, but sometimes they become blocked with fluid, which leads to a discharge (which may be bloody or non-bloody) from the nipple. The lining of the ducts can also become ulcerated, which may cause pain. In addition, inflammation or infection may develop in the ducts. Sometimes a lump can be felt, and it is not unusual for the nipple to pull inwards. Duct ectasia is a benign condition, but can sometimes be mistaken for cancer if a hard lump develops around the abnormal duct. Usually duct ectasia does not need treatment, or else it improves with the application of heat or antibiotic drugs. Occasionally the affected duct may need to be surgically removed via an incision at the border of the areola.

Ectopic prolactin synthesis

See pituitary cancer (page 101) and hyperprolactinoma (page 99).

Fibroadenoma

A fibroadenoma is a benign solid lump of tissue which, although very common in young women, can occur at any age. It is commonly believed that fibroadenoma is a result of increased sensitivity to the female hormone oestrogen. Normally rubbery in texture and often painless, a fibroadenoma is smooth to the touch and moves easily under the skin. It is often called a 'breast mouse', and it is not unusual for more than one to be present.

Fibroadenomas between 1 and 3 cm in diameter are described as *common* fibroadenomas, those that grow to more than 5 cm in diameter are termed *giant* fibroadenomas, and those found in teenage girls are known as *juvenile* fibroadenomas. They usually remain the same size, although some get smaller and some eventually disappear over time. Occasionally fibroadenomas get larger, and this may be more noticeable during pregnancy and breastfeeding. If the lump gets larger or is painful, it can be removed surgically.

Fibrocystic breast disease

Fibrocystic breast disease is defined as common benign changes involving the tissues of the breast. The condition is so commonly found in normal breasts that it is believed to be a normal variant. The cause is not completely understood, but the changes are believed to be associated with ovarian hormones, as the condition usually subsides with the menopause, and breast tissue may vary in consistency during the menstrual cycle.

The incidence is estimated to be over 60% of all women. It is common in women between the ages of 30 and 50 years, and rare in post-menopausal women. The incidence is lower in women who are taking oral contraceptives. The risk factors may include family history and diet (e.g. excessive dietary fat, high caffeine intake), although these are controversial.

Symptoms

- A dense, irregular and bumpy 'cobblestone' consistency in the breast tissue, usually more marked in the outer upper quadrants.

- Breast discomfort that is persistent, or that occurs sporadically.
- A feeling of fullness in the breast(s).
- Dull, heavy pain and tenderness.
- Premenstrual tenderness and swelling.
- A reduction in breast discomfort after each menstrual period.
- Changes in nipple sensation, and itching.

Treatment

- Self-care may include restricting dietary fat intake and eliminating caffeine from the diet.
- It is important to perform a breast self-examination monthly, and to wear a well-fitting bra to provide good breast support.
- Oral contraceptives may be prescribed because they often decrease the symptoms.

Galactocele

A galactocele is a milk cyst (a clogged milk duct), usually associated with child-birth. It occurs in both breastfeeding and non-breastfeeding mothers.

Granulomatous lobular mastitis

This is a condition that affects young women of childbearing age, and is characterised by the formation of multiple peripheral abscesses in the breast. There may be large areas of infection. It is a chronic inflammatory condition which may be due to TB, sarcoidosis, Wegener's granulomatosis or mammary duct ectasia. It is difficult to treat, as the condition tends to recur. Therefore extensive surgery should be avoided.

Hyperprolactinaemia

Prolactin levels are normally high during pregnancy and lactation. Abnormally high levels of prolactin may be caused by a prolactin-secreting pituitary tumour or by a non-secreting pituitary tumour that prevents dopamine (which inhibits prolactin release) from reaching normal prolactin-producing cells. Raised prolactin levels are also sometimes found in hypothyroidism and PCOS, and are associated with a number of different classes of drugs, notably dopamine-receptor antagonists (e.g. metoclopramide, domperidone and the phenothiazines). The behaviour of prolactin-secreting tumours is determined by their size at presentation. In women, absent periods and/or inappropriate production of breast milk allow the diagnosis to be made early.

See pituitary cancer (page 101) and hyperprolactinoma (page 99).

Intraductal papilloma

An intraductal papilloma is a benign wart-like lump that forms within a duct just behind the areola. There may be a small lump and/or a discharge of clear, sticky or bloodstained fluid from the nipple. Intraductal papillomas can be present in both breasts at the same time, and are sometimes discovered following breast surgery. Women nearing the menopause are more likely to have a single intra-ductal papilloma, whereas younger women often have more than one.

Diagnosis

This is made on the basis of triple assessment:

1   breast examination
2   mammogram or ultrasound
3   FNA.

Some clinics perform a core biopsy instead, which involves the removal of tissue samples rather than cells. Women under 35 years of age are usually given a USS rather than a mammogram, as younger breast tissue is denser and produces a less detailed mammogram. In some cases it may not be possible to confirm the diagnosis by triple assessment, and a small operation may be needed to remove the affected duct or ducts. If there is a nipple discharge rather than a lump, a sample is taken and examined under the microscope to confirm the diagnosis.

Treatment

Once the diagnosis has been confirmed, treatment is not always necessary. However, if a lump can be felt and/or the discharge persists, the affected duct or ducts can be removed.

Useful resources

www.breastcancercare.org.uk

Lax cyst

Breast cysts are benign fluid-filled sacs that develop within the breast tissue. They normally affect women over the age of 35 years who have not reached the menopause. However, they are also found in women who are taking hormone replacement therapy (HRT) after the menopause.

Cysts can be present in both breasts, and they may become larger, tender and painful just before a period. Cysts can also be present without any symptoms, and they are sometimes found by chance when tests are done for another reason.

If the cyst is large or does not go away on its own, the fluid can be drawn off with a fine needle and syringe. Once the fluid has been removed, the cyst usually disappears. The fluid that is drawn off will only be sent to the laboratory for testing if it is bloodstained, as there is a small risk that this may be a sign of breast cancer.

Cysts can recur, and this happens in about 30% of cases. The treatment will be the same each time, and there is no need for any further investigations. If a cyst continues to refill, a surgical biopsy may be offered to remove it.

Lipoma

A lipoma is a soft fatty lump. It is a benign growth composed of fat cells that clump together. Lipomas can occur in any part of the body where there are fat cells. They often form in the fatty tissue under the skin. These are also the most noticeable ones, as they look and feel like soft, dome-shaped lumps under the skin. They vary from the size of a pea to several centimetres in diameter. The most common sites for development of lipomas are on the shoulders, the chest and the back, but other areas of the skin can develop lipomas. Anyone can develop a lipoma at any age. In themselves, lipomas are not serious, and most of them cause no symptoms or problems. They grow very slowly. Sometimes a lipoma under the skin can be unsightly if it grows to several centimetres in diameter. Lipomas can be surgically removed, but are generally left alone unless they are causing problems by exerting pressure on other structures.

Mastitis

Mastitis is inflammation of the breast. Most cases of mastitis occur in breast-feeding mothers, although the condition can also occur in women who are not breastfeeding. It is sometimes caused by an infection spreading from another part of the body, or by bacteria entering the breast via cracked or pierced nipples. Usually mastitis is an acute condition, but in rare cases it can be chronic.

Symptoms

The main symptoms are as follows:

- high temperature.
- redness, swelling and hardening of the affected breast.
- severe pain when the breast is pressed.
- enlarged and tender lymph nodes in the armpit.
- general aches and pains, and headache.

The following symptoms are sometimes seen:

- a cracked nipple or a break in the skin
- if the woman is breastfeeding or expressing milk, the breast becomes engorged because it is not draining properly
- the baby may not want to feed from the affected breast, because the taste of the milk has changed.

Treatment

Mild cases of mastitis can be relieved by adopting the following simple measures at home:

- hot showers or hot compresses
- continuing breastfeeding on the affected side

- after each feed, ensuring that the breast is empty and any remaining milk is expressed
- giving the baby the affected breast first, to ensure that it is completely drained
- using painkillers such as ibuprofen or paracetamol for any pain.

Severe mastitis requires urgent treatment with antibiotics. If the mastitis develops further to form an abscess, the latter will need to be surgically opened and drained.

Male factor infertility

- **Azoospermia**

- **Hypogonadotropic hypogonadism**

- **Mucus hostility**

- **Sperm dysfunction**

Male reproductive organs

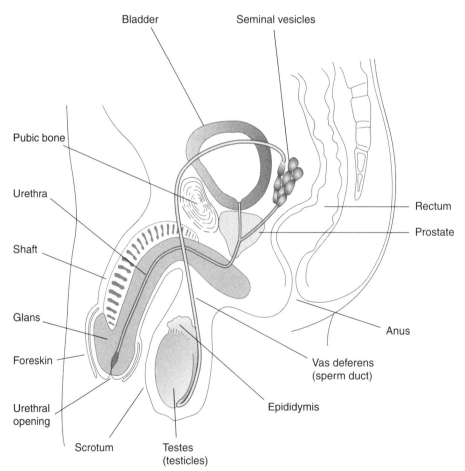

Figure 5   Male reproductive organs: side view.

Azoospermia

Azoospermia is defined as a complete lack of sperm in the ejaculate. This rare condition is sometimes symptomatic of testicular disease or blockage. Often the cause of testicular disease is unknown, but it may be related to mumps or to genetic disorders such as Y-chromosome deletions. Azoospermia is also symptomatic of Klinefelter's syndrome. A lack of sperm in the semen can indicate a blockage in the vas deferens. A vasography can be used to test for blockages.

Treatment

- A testicular biopsy can retrieve sperm to be used in *in-vitro* fertilisation (IVF) or intracytoplasmic sperm injection (ICSI).
- Surgery may be used to correct a blockage.
- Donor sperm may be an option if the condition cannot be corrected.

Hypogonadotropic hypogonadism

Hypogonadotropic hypogonadism describes absent or decreased function of the male testis or the female ovary (the gonads). It is due to the absence of the gonadal stimulating pituitary hormones FSH and LH, and is also known as Kallmann's syndrome.

An area of the brain called the hypothalamus secretes gonadotropin-releasing hormone (GnRH), which stimulates the pituitary gland. In response to this hormone, the pituitary gland secretes FSH and LH. These hormones in turn stimulate the ovaries and testes to secrete hormones that are responsible for normal sexual development in puberty. Any disruption to this cascade causes a deficiency of the sex hormones and halts normal sexual maturation.

Failure of the hypothalamus is most commonly a result of Kallmann's syndrome, which is an inherited disorder. Failure of the pituitary may also result from empty sella syndrome, pituitary tumours and head injuries.

Symptoms

- Lack of development at puberty, incomplete development or significant delay of pubertal development.
- Prepubertal testicular size in adolescence.
- Absence of secondary sexual development (e.g. pubic, facial and underarm hair).
- Short stature may be associated with some forms of hypogonadism.
- Anosmia (inability to smell).

Diagnosis

- Serum hormone levels.
- GnRH stimulation test (measuring hormone levels after stimulation by injected hormones).
- MRI of the head.

Treatment

Treatment depends on the source of the defect, and may include any of the following:

- intramuscular (IM) testosterone or slow-release testosterone skin patch
- oestrogen and progesterone pills
- GnRH injections.

Mucus hostility

The cervical mucus is a jelly-like substance produced by minute glands in the cervical canal. It changes in consistency and composition with the menstrual cycle. Just before ovulation and under the effect of the hormone oestrogen it becomes very watery and copious to allow the sperm to swim through it. After ovulation and under the effect of progesterone, the mucus becomes thick and sticky, which renders it impenetrable to the sperm. Once the sperm are in the mucus, they can remain there for several days. Thus the mucus acts as a sperm reservoir.

Cervical mucus hostility is the inability of sperm to penetrate the cervical mucus. The mucus is too thick and sticky, and there is not enough of it to allow sperm to swim through. This may be due to poor oestrogen stimulation of the cervical glands, possibly due to anovulation, or to poorly functioning cervical glands due to infection or damage caused by surgery, as may occur after cone biopsy. The mucus may contain antisperm antibodies.

The significance of cervical mucus hostility is disputed among infertility specialists.

Sperm dysfunction

In sperm dysfunction there is a normal semen analysis but the sperm either lack or have a defective fertilising capacity, resulting in either complete failure of fertilisation or poor fertilisation of the eggs in IVF. This accounts for 3–6% of male infertility.

Other conditions

Addison's disease – a condition in which insufficient cortisol and other hormones are produced by the adrenal glands. Various symptoms develop if the cortisol concentration becomes too low, and a very low cortisol level can be life-threatening. The classic feature of primary Addison's disease is hyper-pigmentation of the skin on the knuckles, elbows and knees, as well as on new scars, nipples, palmer creases and pressure areas (e.g. buttocks, and the skin under brassiere or belt) and mucous membranes. Other symptoms can include anorexia, weight loss, abdominal pain and tiredness. Treatment is with replacement hormone tablets, which are taken every day.

Adenomyosis – the presence of ectopic endometrial tissue within the myometrium. It is associated with any kind of uterine trauma that may break down the barrier between the endometrium and the myometrium, such as Caesarean section, tubal ligation, any pregnancy, and termination of pregnancy.

Alopecia areata – hair loss or baldness. There are several different causes and patterns of alopecia. Alopecia areata is one type. It is thought to be an auto-immune disease.

Alzheimer's disease – a progressive brain disorder that gradually destroys the affected individual's memory and ability to learn, reason, make judgements, communicate and carry out daily activities. As the disease progresses, the individual may also experience changes in personality and behaviour, such as anxiety, suspiciousness or agitation, as well as delusions or hallucinations.

Anaemia – a deficiency of red blood cells, which can lead to a lack of oxygen-carrying ability of the bloodstream, causing abnormal tiredness and other symptoms.

Anorexia nervosa – a psychophysiological condition, mainly occurring in girls and young women, that is characterised by inability or refusal to eat. The main clinical features of the condition are a reduction in body weight, with a body mass index below $17.5 \, \text{kg/m}^2$, an intense desire to remain thin, and amenorrhoea in females.

Aplasia cutis – a rare disorder with a complicated pattern of inheritance, in which babies are born with the absence of certain layer(s) of skin, most often on the scalp, but also on the trunk and/or arms and legs. The affected area is typically covered with a thin transparent membrane. The skull and/or underlying areas may be visible and abnormally developed. Aplasia cutis congenita may be the primary disorder, or it may occur in association with other underlying disorders.

Appendicitis – a condition characterised by inflammation of the appendix. Mild cases may resolve without treatment, but most cases require removal of the inflamed appendix by either laparotomy or laparoscopy. If left untreated, the mortality rate is high, mainly due to peritonitis and shock.

Asperger's syndrome – a neurobiological disorder characterised by a pattern of behaviours in individuals who have normal intelligence and language development, but who also exhibit autistic-like behaviours and marked deficiencies in social and communication skills.

Autism – a developmental disability that affects the way in which an individual communicates with and relates to people around them. Children and adults with autism have difficulty with everyday social interactions. Their ability to develop friendships is generally limited, as is their capacity to understand the emotional state of other people.

Behçet's disease – a chronic condition caused by disturbances in the body's immune system. This system, which normally protects the body against infections by producing controlled inflammation, becomes overactive and produces unpredictable outbreaks of exaggerated inflammation. This abnormal inflammation affects blood vessels (usually the small ones). As a result, symptoms occur wherever there is an area of inflammation, and can develop anywhere where there is a blood supply.

Bilharzia (schistosomiasis) – a disease caused by parasitic worms. Fresh water becomes contaminated by *Schistosoma* eggs when infected people urinate or defecate in the water. The eggs hatch, and if certain species of snail are present in the water, the parasite grows and develops inside them. The parasite then leaves the snail and enters the water, where it can survive for about 48 hours. *Schistosoma* – parasites can penetrate the skin of people who are wading, swimming, bathing or washing in contaminated water. Within a few weeks, worms grow inside the blood vessels of the body and produce eggs. Some of these eggs travel to the bladder or intestines and are passed into the urine or stool. Within days of becoming infected, a rash or itchy skin may develop. Fever, chills, cough and muscle aches can begin within 1 to 2 months of infection. Most people have no symptoms during this early phase of infection. *Schistosoma* – eggs travel to the liver or pass into the intestine or bladder. Rarely, eggs are found in the brain or spinal cord, and can cause seizures, paralysis or spinal cord inflammation. If people are repeatedly infected for many years, the parasite can damage the liver, intestines, lungs and bladder. Symptoms of schistosomiasis are caused by the body's reaction to the eggs produced by the parasitic worms, not by the worms themselves.

Bornholm disease – a viral infection that affects the intercostal muscles. The lining of the lungs, known as the pleura, may also be affected. This disease is also known as epidemic pleurodynia. Sudden onset of fever and pain occurs around 4 days after infection. During this incubation period, flu-like symptoms may occur. Pain is usually experienced in the chest or upper abdomen.

Bowel obstruction – a mechanical blockage of the intestines that prevents the normal transit of the products of digestion.

Chronic renal failure – a slowly progressive loss of renal function over a period of months or years, defined as an abnormally low glomerular filtration rate, which is usually determined indirectly by the creatinine level in blood serum.

Coeliac disease – a condition of the small intestine in which gluten, a substance found in wheat, barley and rye, reacts with the small bowel, causing damage by activating the immune system to attack the delicate lining of the bowel which is responsible for absorbing nutrients and vitamins.

Condylomata acuminata – genital warts.

Crohn's disease – a chronic inflammatory disease that causes stomach pains, diarrhoea and weight loss. The disease is characterised by periods of activity and remissions. It typically affects the ileum or the colon, but can affect any part of the digestive system. The affected areas become red and swollen, and ulceration may occur. As the ulcers heal, the formation of scar tissue makes the intestine increasingly narrow, leading to obstruction. There is no cure for Crohn's disease, but the symptoms can be treated and the periods of remission can be prolonged for up to several years. The cause of the condition is unknown, but it tends to be more common in relatives of patients with Crohn's disease.

Cushing's syndrome – a hormonal disorder caused by prolonged exposure of the body's tissues to high levels of the hormone cortisol. The symptoms vary, but in most cases there is upper body obesity, a rounded face, increased fat around the neck, and thinning of the arms and legs. Other symptoms affect the skin, which becomes fragile and thin, bruises easily and heals poorly. Purplish-pink stretch marks may appear on the abdomen, thighs, buttocks, arms and breasts. The bones are weakened, and routine activities such as bending, lifting or getting up from a chair may lead to backache and fractures of the rib and spinal column. In most cases there is severe fatigue, muscular weakness, high blood pressure and high blood sugar levels. Irritability, anxiety and depression are common. Women usually have excess hair growth on their face, neck, chest, abdomen and thighs, and their menstrual periods may become irregular or stop.

   Many people develop the symptoms of Cushing's syndrome because they are taking glucocorticoid hormones such as prednisolone for asthma, rheumatoid arthritis, lupus or other inflammatory diseases, or for immunosuppression after transplantation. Others develop Cushing's syndrome because the body is over-producing cortisol due to hormone gland disruption.

Cystitis – inflammation of the bladder.

Darier's disease – a rare inherited skin condition in which the skin in certain areas develops numerous small brownish warty bumps. The disease runs in certain families, being inherited in a pattern known as *dominant inheritance* – which means that there is a 1 in 2 (50:50) chance that each child of an affected parent will inherit the condition. It affects both men and women, and is not contagious or due to an allergy. In normal skin, the skin cells are held together like bricks cemented in a wall. However, in Darier's disease the sticky junctions that hold the skin cells together are not formed properly, and the skin may become scaly or lumpy or even form blisters. The first signs of the condition usually appear somewhere between the ages of 6 and 20 years. Small brownish roughened bumps develop on the skin. The severity of the condition varies considerably and is unpredictable. The rash often occurs on the chest, neck or upper back initially, but warty bumps may occur on any part of the body.

Dermatosis – any disorder of the skin.

Diabetes mellitus – a disorder that occurs when the level of glucose in the blood becomes higher than normal. There are two main types of diabetes:

- *type 1 diabetes*, in which the pancreas stops making insulin. The illness and symptoms develop quickly (over days or weeks) because the level of insulin in the bloodstream becomes very low. The disorder usually first develops in childhood or young adulthood
- *type 2 diabetes*, in which the illness and symptoms tend to develop gradually (over weeks or months), because in this type of diabetes the pancreas still makes insulin. However, diabetes develops for one of the following reasons:
  – not enough insulin is made for the body's needs
  – the body's cells do not use insulin properly (a condition known as insulin resistance), so more insulin is needed to keep the blood glucose level down
  – a combination of the above two reasons.

Discoid lupus erythematosus – a chronic skin condition characterised by inflammation and scarring skin lesions on the face, ears and scalp and sometimes on other body areas. These lesions develop as an inflamed growth with scaling and a wart-like appearance. The central area may appear lighter in colour, surrounded by an area that is darker than the normal skin. A small percentage of cases develop disease of the internal organs, which can cause systemic symptoms.

Diverticulosis – a condition characterised by the presence of diverticula. In many people there are small pouches in the colon that bulge outward through weak spots. Each pouch is called a diverticulum (diverticula in the plural). When the pouches become infected or inflamed, the condition is called diverticulitis. This occurs in 10–25% of people with diverticulosis. Diverticulosis and diverticulitis are also known as diverticular disease. The commonest symptom of diverticulitis is abdominal pain, and the commonest sign is tenderness around the left side of the lower abdomen. If infection is the cause, fever, nausea, vomiting, chills, cramping and constipation may occur as well. The severity of symptoms depends on the extent of the infection and complications. Diverticulitis can lead to bleeding, infections, perforations or tears, or blockages. These complications always require treatment to prevent them from progressing and causing serious illness.

Dyspepsia – this is a catch-all term that includes a variety of digestive problems, such as stomach discomfort, trapped gas, bloating, belching, appetite loss and nausea.

Dysplasia (Latin for 'bad form') – an abnormality in the appearance of cells indicative of an early step towards transformation into neoplasia – that is, a preneoplastic or pre-cancerous change. This abnormal growth is restricted to the epithelial layer, and does not invade the deeper tissue. Although dysplasia may regress spontaneously, persistent lesions must be removed by surgery, chemical burning/topical medication, heat burning/diathermy, laser treatment or cryotherapy.

Erythema multiforme – an allergic reaction that has many different causes. It often starts as a red rash on the palms, soles and the backs of the hands. In severe cases it can spread to the trunk, face and mouth. As the skin lesions age, they often resemble small targets with purple to dusky centres surrounded by red rings. The condition can be associated with fever, aching muscles and generally feeling unwell. The causes of erythema multiforme include allergic reactions to viral, bacterial and fungal infections, sensitivity to food or drugs, and immunisations. The condition may also occur in association with other disorders.

Factor XI deficiency – an inherited bleeding disorder. Factor XI is a trace protein in the blood. It is produced by the liver, and plays a role in the coagulation cascade – that is, the chain reaction that is set in motion when a blood vessel becomes injured. Factor XI appears to aid the activation of factor IX, another blood protein that is important in the clotting process.

Fanconi's syndrome – impairment of the proximal tubular function of the kidney. It may be inherited or arise spontaneously. This impairment causes certain compounds (glucose, amino acids, uric acid and phosphate), which should be transferred to the bloodstream via the kidneys, to be excreted in the urine instead, resulting in growth failure, decreased bone mineralisation and abnormal bone mineralisation.

Folliculitis – inflammation of a number of hair follicles of the skin. Most cases of folliculitis are due to infection with a bacterium called *Staphylococcus aureus*. The affected hair follicles swell to form small pus-filled pimples. They occur in crops, usually at sites where hair follicles are damaged by friction or shaving, or where there is blockage of the follicle.

Frey's syndrome – an autonomic disorder characterised by excessive sweating of the skin on the forehead, upper lip, perioral region or sternum subsequent to gustatory stimuli. The condition may develop after trauma to the parotid gland, in association with parotid neoplasms, or following surgical removal of the latter.

Furuncle – a common skin infection involving an entire hair follicle and the adjacent subcutaneous tissue, usually caused by *Staphylococcus* – bacteria. Damage to the hair follicle allows these bacteria to enter deeper into the tissues of the follicle and the subcutaneous tissue. Furuncles may occur in the hair follicles anywhere on the body, but they most commonly occur on the face, neck, armpit, buttocks and thighs. They may be single or multiple.

Granuloma inguinale – a sexually transmitted infection that is rarely seen in western countries. It causes surface destruction and granuloma formation in the skin and subcutaneous tissue. The disease is commonly found in tropical and subtropical areas such as South-East India, Guyana and New Guinea. The infection is twice as common in men as in women, with most cases occurring in individuals aged 20 to 40 years. The disease is seldom seen in children or the elderly. It is thought that anal intercourse, rather than vaginal intercourse, is the most frequent route of infection; about 50% of infected men and women have lesions in the anal area. Antibiotic treatment is indicated.

Haemochromatosis – a hereditary disease characterised by impaired processing by the body of dietary iron, which causes iron to accumulate in a number of body tissues, eventually causing organ dysfunction.

Haemorrhoids (also known as piles) – varicosities (swelling and inflammation of veins) in the rectum and anus.

Hepatitis – inflammation of the liver.

Hernia – a protrusion of a tissue, structure or part of an organ through the muscular tissue or the membrane that normally encloses it.

Hives (also known as urticaria) – a relatively common form of allergic reaction that causes raised red skin welts.

Hydradenitis supparativa – a chronic and relapsing disorder of the apocrine sweat glands, which most commonly occurs in women. Deep-seated inflammatory nodules form in the axilla, groin, pubic region and perineum. It is an androgen-dependent disorder caused by keratinous material occluding the sweat pores.

Hypocalcaemia – a low serum calcium concentration. Calcium is a component of bones and teeth, and is also essential for normal blood clotting and muscle and nerve functioning. Hypocalcaemia can have a number of causes, including hypoparathyroidism, failure to produce dihydroxyvitamin D, low levels of plasma magnesium, and inadequate dietary intake of calcium or vitamin D. Hypoparathyroidism is characterised by the failure of the parathyroid gland to make parathyroid hormone. This hormone controls and maintains plasma calcium levels. Magnesium is required for parathyroid hormone to play its part in maintaining plasma calcium levels.

Hypokalaemia – a low serum potassium concentration, relating to regulation of both the internal balance between intra- and extracellular fluids and the external balance determining the total body potassium level. This is achieved by the kidney, mainly under the control of the hormone aldosterone, which is secreted by the adrenal glands. Most cases of hypokalaemia are a result of either diuretic consumption or loss of gastrointestinal fluids due to persistent vomiting, chronic diarrhoea or laxative abuse. In the case of loss due to vomiting, the cause of the condition is not direct loss of potassium, but loss of chloride resulting in high levels of aldosterone and inhibiting reabsorption of potassium from the kidney tubules. In diarrhoea, loss of bicarbonate may cause metabolic acidosis, which causes a shift of potassium into the cells so that the serum concentration may not reflect total potassium levels.

Irritable bowel syndrome – a common functional bowel disorder, the main symptoms of which are abdominal bloating and multiple areas of abdominal pain, the pain often being relieved on defecation. There may also be changes in bowel habit. The cause is not known. An organic trigger, such as bacterial gastro-enteritis, is seen in some patients. However, there is undoubtedly a psychological component. Management consists of explanation, fibre supplements, antispasmodics and antidepressants.

Jaundice – a yellowing of the skin, sclera (the whites of the eyes) and mucous membranes caused by increased levels of bilirubin in the body. When red blood cells die, the haem in their haemoglobin is converted to bilirubin in the spleen and in the Kupffer cells in the liver. The bilirubin is processed by the liver, enters the bile and is eventually eliminated in the faeces. Thus disruption of any of these processes can cause jaundice.

Kallmann's syndrome – the occurrence of hypothalamic gonadotropin-releasing hormone deficiency and impairment of olfactory sensation (hyposmia or anosmia). It is inherited as an X-linked or autosomal recessive disorder with greater penetrance in the male. Gonadotropin deficiency is due to failure of embryonic migration of GnRH-secreting neurons from their site of origin in the nose. The same defect affects the olfactory neurons, resulting in olfactory bulb aplasia. More than 50% of affected patients have associated somatic stigmata, most commonly nerve deafness, colour blindness, midline craniofacial deformities such as cleft palate or harelip, and renal abnormalities. Female patients may present with primary amenorrhoea, and male patients with cryptorchidism.

Kidney cyst – a round swelling in the kidney, with a very thin, clear wall, and usually filled with watery fluid. The kidney is composed of blood vessels which carry blood to tiny filters. Each filter is connected to a tube. There are about a million filter-and-tube units in each kidney. A cyst occurs when a single tube expands, often becoming quite large. The exact cause of the swelling of the tube is not known. Some cysts are normal, but there is a possibility that they can interfere with kidney function.

Kidney stones – solid crystals formed from minerals that have separated from the urine. They are found inside the kidneys or ureters, and typically leave the body in the urine stream. If they grow relatively large before being passed, obstruction of a ureter and distension with urine can cause severe pain, most commonly experienced in the flank, lower abdomen and groin.

Kleinfelter's syndrome – a condition caused by chromosome non-disjunction in males, in which affected individuals have a pair of X chromosomes instead of just one. It is associated with an increased risk of developing some medical conditions. XXY males are almost always sterile, and some degree of language impairment may be present. In adults, possible characteristics vary widely and range from few to no signs, to a lanky, youthful body type and facial appearance, or a rounded body type with some degree of gynaecomastia (increased breast tissue). The most severe cases are also associated with an increased risk of breast cancer, pulmonary disease, varicose veins and osteoporosis – risks that are shared with women.

Laurence–Moon–Biedl syndrome – an autosomal recessive condition characterised by mental retardation, retinitis pigmentosa, hypogonadism, spastic paraplegia, obesity, polydactyly, cataract, squint and renal abnormalities.

Leukoplakia – a condition of the mouth that is characterised by the formation of white leathery spots on the mucous membranes of the tongue and inside the mouth. In most cases the cause is unknown, but many are related to tobacco use and chronic irritation. A small proportion of cases, particularly those involving the floor of the mouth or the lower surface of the tongue, are associated with a risk of cancer.

Lichen planus – a condition that affects the skin, causing an itchy rash that typically consists of small, reddish-purple bumps (papules). The bumps are usually shiny and flat-topped, and range from the size of a pinhead to about 1 cm in diameter.

Lichen sclerosus – an uncommon skin condition that affects either the vulva or the foreskin and the end of the penis. In women, small 'pearly-white' spots typically develop on the vulva. The spots are usually itchy and shiny. In about 3 in 10 cases, the skin around the anus is also affected. Sometimes only the skin around the anus is affected. The itch and irritation usually become persistent and distressing. The itching tends to be worse at night, and can disturb sleep. Sometimes soreness rather than itching is the main symptom. Lichen sclerosus is a skin condition only, and does not extend into the vagina or the anus. Over time the white spots may become larger and join together. The whole vulva and/or anal area may then become white, and is more fragile than normal. The fragile skin may become damaged, inflamed, raw and prone to painful splitting and cracking, and it may become painful to have sex. If the anal skin is affected, passing a bowel motion may cause pain or splitting of the skin. If the condition is left untreated, over months or years the vulva may atrophy. Scarring may develop, and this may cause fusion of the labia, which can narrow the entrance to the vagina, making it difficult to have sex. In addition, thrush and other infections tend to be more common if the vulva is sore or cracked.

In men, white spots develop on the foreskin and the end of the penis. These may itch and be sore. This may progress to cause scarring, which may lead to difficulty in retracting the foreskin and passing urine. Erections may become painful. The anal skin is rarely affected in men.

The cause of lichen sclerosus is not known. There is some inflammation in the dermis layer of the skin, which causes changes to the structure of the affected skin, although it is not clear why this happens. It is possible that lichen sclerosus is an autoimmune disease.

Lymphogranuloma venereum (LGV) – a sexually transmitted infection caused by *Chlamydia trachomatis*. It is endemic in tropical regions of Africa, India, South-East Asia, South America and the Caribbean, with men more commonly affected than women, mainly between the ages of 20 and 30 years.

The disease has three stages:

1   an asymptomatic ulcer which resolves rapidly
2   an inguinal syndrome, which develops between 1 week and 6 months later, with adenopathy (enlarged and painful lymph nodes) and bubo (a greatly enlarged lymph node that is tender and painful, particularly in the groin or armpit) development. There is often systemic illness and malaise
3   a regional abscess or fistula, resulting in regional strictures (e.g. rectal strictures).

Diagnosis is by serology and intradermal skin test with LGV antigen (Frei's test). The condition remits spontaneously, but can be treated with antibiotics.

Microsporum canis – a fungal skin infection.

Migraine – a condition that causes episodes of severe headache, and often other symptoms such as nausea or vomiting. For most people who have migraine, attacks occur for no apparent reason. However, there may be triggers for migraine attacks in some individuals for example, certain foods, wine or stress. Some women have migraines before or during periods. The actual cause of the migraine is thought to be a fall in the blood level of the hormone oestrogen just before a period. It is not a low level of oestrogen that is the trigger, but rather the change from one level to another.

The strict definition of menstrual migraine is migraine that starts any time from 2 days before to 3 days after the first day of a period, and that occurs around the time of most (or all) periods.

Mondor's disease – thrombophlebitis of the superficial veins of the breast or chest wall. The main symptom is acute pain, frequently following trauma.

Nephritis – inflammation of the kidney.

Pancreatitis – inflammation of the pancreas.

Parkinson's disease – a progressive neurological condition that affects movement of the body.

Peptic ulcer disease – an ulcer of the gastrointestinal tract. Most ulcers are now known to be associated with *Helicobacter pylori*, a spiral-shaped bacterium that lives in the acidic environment of the stomach. Ulcers can also be caused or worsened by drugs such as aspirin and other NSAIDs. About 4% of gastric ulcers are caused by a malignant tumour, which is one reason to be vigilant about detecting them. Duodenal ulcers are generally non-malignant.

Postviral syndrome (also known as chronic fatigue syndrome, myalgic encephalitis or fibromyalgia) – an illness characterised by a number of symptoms similar to those of severe flu. The characteristic feature is fatigue which persists for more than 6 months and for which no other cause can be found. It may follow an infection such as flu or tonsillitis. The fatigue affects both mental and physical activity, and is not relieved by rest. Other symptoms may include sweating, shivering, feeling cold, headaches and nausea. Bowel problems such as diarrhoea or constipation can occur. Visual problems and generalised aches and pains, especially in muscles or joints, may occur. Affected patients complain of poor memory and difficulty in concentrating. All of these symptoms may vary from day to day and are often made worse by minimal physical or mental effort. Mood swings may occur, and the patient may feel tearful and depressed.

Prader–Willi syndrome – a genetic syndrome caused by a disorder of chromosome 15. The main features are obesity, cognitive impairment, behaviour problems, poor muscle tone and hypogonadism.

Psoriasis – a common skin condition which typically causes the development of patches of red, scaly skin. The severity of the condition varies widely. Once an individual develops psoriasis it tends to recur throughout life. The exact cause is unknown.

Pyelonephritis – an ascending urinary tract infection that has reached the pyelum (pelvis) of the kidney.

Pyuria – the presence of white blood cells in the urine, usually a symptom of urinary tract infection.

Reiter's syndrome – a disorder consisting of a triad of symptoms, namely urethritis, conjunctivitis and seronegative arthritis. Two broad subtypes are recognised – a genital form related to sexual activity, and an enteric form related to gastrointestinal infection. Reiter's syndrome is the result of a genetically determined pathological immune response to an infectious agent. The following agents are implicated:

- genital form – *Chlamydia*, gonorrhoea
- enteric form – *Salmonella, Yersinia, Shigella, Campylobacter.*

Rhesus factor (also known as Rh factor) – the presence or absence of a particular protein (originally discovered while studying Rhesus monkeys), which is present in the blood of some people but not others. If a person's blood does contain the protein, it is said to be Rh positive (Rh+). If it does not contain the protein it is described as Rh negative (Rh−).

This Rh factor is connected to blood type. For example, blood may be AB+, which means that it is type AB blood with a positive Rh factor, or it may be O−, which means that it is type O blood with a negative Rh factor.

It is particularly important for expectant mothers to know their blood's Rh factor. Occasionally, a baby will inherit an Rh-positive blood type from its father while the mother has an Rh-negative blood type. The baby's life could then be in great danger if the mother's Rh-negative blood attacks the baby's Rh-positive blood. If this happens, an exchange transfusion may save the baby's life. The baby's blood can be exchanged for new blood which matches that of the mother.

Ringworm – a fungal skin infection.

Scleroderma morphea – (from the Greek term for 'hard skin') a group of autoimmune diseases in which there is increased fibroblast activity, resulting in abnormal growth of connective tissue, which leads to vascular damage and fibrosis. It may be either localised or systemic.

Seborrhoeic dermatitis – inflammation of areas of the skin that have many sebaceous glands, such as the side of the nose, the forehead and the scalp. Seborrhoeic dermatitis is a harmless and common condition.

Shingles (also known as herpes zoster) – a painful, blistering rash caused by the chickenpox (varicella) virus, which affects only a limited area of skin. Shingles only occurs if an individual has previously had chickenpox, after which the virus lies dormant in the nerves. Shingles occurs when the virus is revitalised in one particular nerve to the skin. This explains the way in which it only affects a clearly demarcated band of skin. Usually the cause is a decrease in the body's natural resistance, which may be due to other infections, stress, being generally run down, or occasionally when the body's immune defences are affected by certain drugs or other immune deficiencies.

Sickle-cell anaemia – an inherited condition in which affected individuals have sickle haemoglobin (HbS), which is different from the normal haemoglobin (HbA). When sickle haemoglobin gives up its oxygen to the tissues, the haemoglobin molecules stick together to form long rods inside the red blood cells. As a result, these cells become rigid and sickle-shaped. Normal red blood cells can bend and flex easily but, because of their shape, sickled red blood cells cannot squeeze through small blood vessels as easily, and this can lead to blocking of these small vessels, which prevents oxygen from reaching the tissues where it is needed. This in turn can lead to anaemia, severe pain and damage to organs.

Skin tag (also known as acrochordon) – a small benign tumour that develops primarily in areas where the skin forms creases, such as the neck, armpits and groin. Skin tags also occur on the face, usually on the eyelids. The surface of acrochordons may be smooth or irregular in appearance. Skin tags are often raised from the surface of the skin on a fleshy stalk known as a *peduncle*. Skin tags are harmless. Their cause is unknown, but there are correlations with age and obesity. They are more common in people with diabetes mellitus.

Spondylosis (cervical/thoracic) (also known as spinal osteoarthritis) – a degenerative disorder that may cause loss of normal spinal structure and function. Although ageing is the primary cause, the location and rate of degeneration varies from one individual to another.

Thoracic outlet syndrome – neurovascular symptoms in the upper extremities due to pressure on the nerves and vessels in the thoracic outlet area. The specific structures that are compressed are usually the nerves of the brachial plexus and occasionally the subclavian artery or subclavian vein.

Tietze's syndrome – a tender, non-suppurative swelling of the costochondral cartilage in the upper costosternal region, which causes chest pain.

Turner's syndrome – a genetic condition that occurs only in female individuals, in which the cells are missing an X chromosome or part of an X chromosome (female cells normally have two X chromosomes). The most common signs and symptoms are short stature, lack of developing ovaries, and infertility.

Ulcerative colitis – a superficial inflammation of the large intestine which results in ulceration and bleeding. The exact cause of ulcerative colitis is unknown. Hereditary, infectious and immunological factors have been proposed as possible causes.

Urinary tract infection (UTI) – infection of the urinary tract. An infection anywhere in the kidneys, ureters, bladder or urethra qualifies as a urinary tract infection.

von Willebrand's disease – an inherited bleeding disorder. Children born with the disease either have low levels of a protein that helps the blood to clot, or else the protein does not function properly.

Tests and procedures

Blood tests

- **Clotting**

- **C-reactive protein**

- **Erythrocyte sedimentation rate**

- **Follicle-stimulating hormone/luteinising hormone**

- **Full blood count**

- **Human chorionic gonadotropin**

- **Liver function**

- **Progesterone**

- **Prolactin**

- **Testosterone**

- **Thyroid function**

- **Urea and electrolytes (U&Es)**

Clotting

The activated partial thromboplastin time (APTT or PTT) is a measure of the functionality of the pathways of the coagulation cascade. The body uses the co-agulation cascade to produce blood clots to seal off injuries to blood vessels and tissues, to prevent further blood loss, and to give the damaged areas time to heal. The cascade consists of a group of coagulation factors. These proteins are activated sequentially along either the extrinsic (tissue-related) or intrinsic (blood vessel-related) pathways. The branches of the pathway then come together into the common pathway, and complete their task with the formation of a stable blood clot. When a person starts bleeding, these three pathways have to work together.

Each component of the coagulation cascade must be functioning properly and must be present in sufficient quantity for normal blood clot formation to occur. If there is an inherited or acquired deficiency of one or more of the factors, or if the factors are functioning abnormally, stable clot formation will be inhibited and excessive bleeding and/or clotting may occur.

The APTT test measures the length of time (in seconds) that it takes for clotting to occur when reagents are added to plasma in a test tube.

The normal range is 26–39 seconds.

C-reactive protein

This test identifies the presence of inflammation, determines its severity and monitors the response to treatment. C-reactive protein (CRP) is a protein made by the liver and secreted into the blood. It is often the first evidence of inflammation or infection in the body. Its concentration in the blood increases within a few hours after the onset of infection or other inflammatory injury. Raised CRP levels in the blood often precede pain, fever or other clinical indicators. The level of CRP can increase 1000-fold in response to inflammation and then drop relatively quickly as soon as the inflammation passes, making it a valuable test for monitoring the effectiveness of treatment.

The normal range is less than 4 mg/l.

Erythrocyte sedimentation rate

The erythrocyte sedimentation rate (ESR) is an indirect measure of the degree of inflammation present in the body. It actually measures the rate of fall (sedimentation) of red blood cells (erythrocytes) in a tall thin tube of blood. The results are expressed as the number of millimetres of clear plasma present at the top of the column after 1 hour. Normally, red cells fall slowly, leaving little clear plasma. However, increased blood levels of certain proteins (such as fibrinogen or immunoglobulins, which are increased in inflammation) cause the red blood cells to fall more rapidly, increasing the ESR. This is an easy, inexpensive, non-specific test that has been used for many years to help to diagnose conditions associated with acute and chronic inflammation, including infections, cancers and auto-immune diseases. ESR is said to be non-specific because an increase in ESR doesn't indicate exactly where the inflammation is located in the body or what is causing it, and also because it can be affected by other conditions as well as inflammation. For this reason, ESR is typically used in conjunction with other tests.

ESR varies widely in different physiological and pathological conditions. It is influenced by age, gender and the presence of anaemia, and must be measured within 2 hours of venepuncture. The normal range varies depending on the technique that is used. The approximate normal range for males is equal to the age in years divided by 2, and for females is equal to the age in years plus 10 divided by 2.

Follicle-stimulating hormone/luteinising hormone

Luteinising hormone (LH) acts together with follicle-stimulating hormone (FSH) in the final stages of maturation of ovarian follicles, stimulating the release of oestrogen from them. At low or constant levels of oestrogen the effect on LH release is negative. However, when oestrogen levels become high as the follicle approaches maturation, positive feedback occurs. The anterior pituitary becomes more responsive to the effect of gonadotropin-releasing hormone, and there is a peak in LH secretion. Ovulation occurs about 9 hours after this peak has been reached.

LH then goes on to promote the formation of the corpus luteum and the secretion of progesterone in the second half of the menstrual cycle.

The high levels of oestrogen, progesterone and inhibin have a negative feedback effect on production of LH by the anterior pituitary during the second half of the menstrual cycle.

FSH:
Normal range (IU/I):
Follicular phase: 2.5–9.7.
Mid-cycle: up to 7.6–19.
Luteal phase: 0.9–5.8.
Post menopause: 12–100.

LH:
Normal range (μ mol/l):
Follicular phase: 0.8–9.0.
Mid-cycle: $\leq$65.
Luteal phase: 0.7–14.5.

Full blood count

The full blood count (FBC) is used as a broad screening test. It is actually a group of tests that examine different components of the blood. The results of the following tests provide the broadest picture of a person's health.

- **White blood cell (WBC) count** measures the total number of white blood cells. Both increases and decreases in WBC can be significant.
  - Normal range is $4–11 \times 10^9$/l.
- **White blood cell differential** measures the different types of white blood cells present. There are five different types of white blood cell, each with its own function in protecting the body from infection. The differential classifies a person's white blood cells into the following types: neutrophils (also known as polymorphs, PMNs or granulocytes), lymphocytes, monocytes, eosinophils and basophils.
  - Normal range: neutrophils, $2.5–7.5 \times 10^9$/l (60–70%); lymphocytes, $1.5–4.0 \times 10^9$/l (25–30%); monocytes, $0.2–0.8 \times 10^9$/l (5–10%); eosinophils, $0.04–0.44 \times 10^9$/l (1–4%); basophils, up to 0.1×10^9/l (up to 1%).
- **Red blood cell (RBC) count** is the number of red blood cells per litre of blood. Both increases and decreases can indicate abnormal conditions.
  - Normal range in males is $4.0–5.9 \times 10^{12}$/l and in females is $3.8–5.2 \times 10^{12}$/l.
- **Haemoglobin** is the amount of oxygen-carrying protein in the blood.
  - Normal range (g/dl) for children:
    at birth: 16.5 (13.5–19.5)
    at 2 weeks: 16.5 (12.5–20.5)
    at 2 months: 11.5 (9–14)

at 6 months: 11.5 (9.5–13.5)
at puberty in males: 13–16
at puberty in females: 12–16.
– Normal range (g/dl) for adults:
males: 13.5–18
females: 11.5–16.5.

- **Haematocrit (also known as packed cell volume or PCV)** is the proportion of space that the red blood cells take up in the blood. It is expressed as a percentage.
    - Normal range (ml) for children:
    at birth: 0.42–0.54
    at 1–3 years: 0.29–0.4
    at 4–10 years: 0.36–0.38.
    - Normal range (ml) for adults:
    males: 0.40–0.54 (41–54%)
    females: 0.35–0.47 (35–47%)

- **Platelet count** is the number of platelets in a given volume of blood. Both increases and decreases in platelet count can indicate abnormal conditions of excess bleeding or clotting. The platelet count is expressed as thousand million platelets per litre.
    - Normal range is $150–400 \times 10^9/l$.

- **Mean platelet volume (MPV)** is a machine-calculated measurement of the average size of a person's platelets. New platelets are larger, and an increased MPV occurs when increased numbers of platelets are being produced. The MPV provides information about platelet production in a person's bone marrow.
    - Normal range is 7.5–11.5 fl.

- **Mean corpuscular volume (MCV)** is a measurement of the average size of the red blood cells (RBCs). The MCV is elevated when RBCs are larger than normal (macrocytic) – for example, in anaemia caused by vitamin B_{12} deficiency. When the MCV is decreased, RBCs are smaller than normal (microcytic) – for example, in iron-deficiency anaemia.
    - Normal range is 80–99 fl.

- **Mean corpuscular haemoglobin (MCH)** is a calculation of the amount of oxygen-carrying haemoglobin inside a person's red blood cells. Since macrocytic RBCs are larger than either normal or microcytic RBCs, they would also tend to have higher MCH values.
    - Normal range is 27–33 pg.

- **Mean corpuscular haemoglobin concentration (MCHC)** is a calculation of the percentage of haemoglobin in the RBCs. Decreased values indicate hypochromasia (decreased oxygen-carrying capacity due to decreased haemoglobin levels inside the cell). Hypochromasia is seen in iron-deficiency anaemia and in thalassaemia.
    - Normal range is 32–36 g/dl.

- **Red cell distribution width (RDW)** is a calculation of the variation in size of the RBCs. In some anaemias, such as pernicious anaemia, the amount of variation (anisocytosis) in RBC size, along with variation in shape (poikilocytosis), is significant.
    - Normal range is 1.5–14.5%.

Human chorionic gonadotropin

Human chorionic gonadotropin (HCG) is a protein produced in the placenta of pregnant women. A pregnancy test is a specific blood or urine test that can detect HCG and confirm pregnancy. This hormone can be detected 10 days after a missed menstrual period, the time period during which the fertilised egg becomes implanted in the woman's uterus. With some methods, HCG can be detected even earlier, at 1 week after conception.

During the early weeks of pregnancy, HCG has an important role in maintaining the functioning of the corpus luteum (the mass of cells that forms from a mature egg). Production of HCG increases steadily during the first trimester (8–10 weeks), peaking at around week 10 after the last menstrual cycle. Levels then fall slowly during the remainder of the pregnancy. HCG is no longer detectable within a few weeks after delivery. It is also produced by some germ-cell tumours, and increased levels are seen in trophoblastic disease.

- The first morning urine should be tested for βHCG.
- *Note:* urinary HCG pregnancy tests do not work after 20 weeks' gestation, and should not be relied upon to exclude pregnancy after a few months of amenorrhoea.
- Less than 50% of tests are positive in extrauterine pregnancies. In cases where an ectopic pregnancy is suspected, the serum HCG level should be requested, as this is 200 times more sensitive.
- A persistently raised serum HCG level of >1000 mlU/ml on consecutive days, in the absence of an intrauterine pregnancy on ultrasound test, is highly suggestive of an ectopic pregnancy.
- A rapidly falling serum HCG level is strongly suggestive of a miscarriage.
- A serum HCG level of <2 indicates that pregnancy is unlikely.
- Women who have repeated false-positive tests should have their serum HCG levels measured in order to check for chorion carcinoma.

Liver function

Liver function is assessed by a range of tests which generally include plasma bilirubin, albumin, and the enzymes alanine transaminase (ALT), aspartate transaminase (AST) and alkaline phosphatase. Individual test results are of less value than consideration of the results as a whole.

Biochemical measures of liver function commonly assess the following:

- hepatic anion transport – principally serum bilirubin
- abnormal protein synthesis:
  - serum albumin – hypoalbuminaemia in chronic liver injury
  - prothrombin time – may be increased because of failure to absorb fat-soluble vitamin K in cholestasis (factors II (prothrombin), VII, IX and X are vitamin K dependent) or due to impaired synthesis of coagulation factors (as above, plus factor V and fibrinogen)
  - serum immunoglobulins – usually increased in chronic liver disease. IgM is predominantly increased in primary biliary cirrhosis, and IgG in chronic autoimmune hepatitis.

- liver enzyme tests:
  - cytoplasmic and mitochondrial enzymes – levels of which are raised when there is liver cell damage. ALT is more liver specific than AST, and its levels rise more than those of AST in early liver cell injury. AST levels rise more in chronic injury.
  - membrane-associated enzymes – alkaline phosphatase and gamma-glutamyltransferase are anchored to the biliary canaliculus. They are raised in biliary outflow obstruction rather than in cases of hepatocellular damage.
- miscellaneous – anti-mitochondrial antibodies (in primary biliary cirrhosis), increased plasma lipids (in cholestasis), serum urea levels (may be reduced in severe hepatic disease).

Serum bilirubin:
Normal range (mol/l) <17.
Total bilirubin: 3–20.
Indirect bilirubin: 0–14.

Albumin:
Normal range is 30–55 g/l (depending on the method used).

Prothrombin time (PT): A standard reference range is not available for this test. Because reference values are dependent on many factors, including patient age, gender, sample population and test method, numerical test results have different meanings in different laboratories. The test result for PT depends on the method used, with results measured in seconds and compared with the average value in healthy individuals. Most laboratories report PT results that have been adjusted to the *international normalised ratio (INR)*. Patients on anticoagulant drugs should have an INR of 2.0–3.0 for basic 'blood-thinning' needs. For some patients who have a high risk of clot formation, the INR needs to be higher (around 2.5–3.5).

Alanine transaminase (ALT):
Normal range is <45 IU/l.

Aspartate transaminase (AST):
Normal range is <50 IU/l.

Alkaline phosphatase:
Normal range is 90–300 IU/l (the level is dependent on the method of assay). In children the levels are two to three times higher than normal values in adults.

Serum immunoglobulins:
Normal range (g/l) (in adults):

- IgA: 1.5–2.5
- IgG: 8–18
- IgM: 0.4–2.9.

Gamma-glutamyltransferase:
Normal range (IU/I):
males: ≤70
females: ≤40.

Progesterone

Since progesterone levels vary predictably throughout the menstrual cycle, multiple measurements can be used to aid recognition and management of some causes of infertility. Progesterone can be measured in order to determine whether or not a woman has ovulated, to determine when ovulation occurred, and to monitor the success of induced ovulation.

In early pregnancy, progesterone measurements may be used, along with human chorionic gonadotropin (HCG) testing, to help to diagnose an ectopic or failing pregnancy (progesterone levels will be lower than expected), although this will not differentiate between the two conditions. Progesterone levels may also be measured throughout a high-risk pregnancy to help to evaluate placental and fetal health. Levels of progesterone will be naturally higher during pregnancies that involve multiples (twins, triplets, etc.) than during those in which there is only one fetus.

Progesterone levels may be monitored in women who have difficulty maintaining a pregnancy, as low levels of the hormone can lead to miscarriage. If a woman is receiving progesterone injections to help to support her early pregnancy, her progesterone levels may be monitored on a regular basis to help to determine the effectiveness of that treatment.

In women who are not pregnant, progesterone levels may be used, along with other tests, to help to determine the cause of abnormal uterine bleeding.

If progesterone levels do not rise and fall on a monthly basis, a woman may not be ovulating or having menstrual periods.

Raised progesterone levels are also occasionally seen in women with luteal ovarian cysts, molar pregnancies or a rare form of ovarian cancer.

Increased progesterone levels are occasionally due to overproduction of progesterone by the adrenal glands. In late pregnancy, low levels of progesterone may be associated with toxaemia and pre-eclampsia.

Plasma progesterone should be measured 7 days before the onset of the next menstrual period. Normal range (nmol/l) is >30 (indicates normal ovulation):

- <16 indicates no ovulation
- 16–30 indicates repeat test
- 0.1–1.0 indicates post menopause.

Prolactin

This is a hormone produced by the anterior pituitary gland. It is released under inhibitory dopaminergic control and stimulatory thyrotropin-releasing hormone (TRH) control. There is increased release of prolactin at night, and in females there is increased release during puberty. Prolactin can be released in response to stress (e.g. exercise), levels are high during pregnancy, and during lactation breastfeeding results in increased release of prolactin.

Prolactin causes breast-milk protein synthesis and excretion in ducts and lobules, and at high levels has a contraceptive effect.

Normal range (MU/l):
males: <20 MU/l
females in follicular phase: <23 or up to 610 MU/l.

Testosterone

Testosterone is a sex steroid hormone. Testosterone stimulates the features of puberty, anabolism and negative feedback on secretion of luteinising hormone by the pituitary gland.

Some testosterone is converted into oestradiol in the liver, adipose tissue and central nervous system. Excessive androgen secretion in women may cause acne, anovulation or hirsutism. Sources include the ovaries, adrenal glands and peripheral tissues, including the skin.

Normal range in women (nmol/l):
pre-menopause: 0.3–2.8
post-menopause: 0.3–1.2.

Thyroid function

The laboratory assessment of hypothyroidism and hyperthyroidism has been simplified by the development of sensitive assays for thyroid-stimulating hormone (TSH), free T_3 and free T_4. Thyrotropin-releasing hormone (TRH) is a tripeptide that is released by the hypothalamus and which stimulates the production of TSH, a polypeptide, from the anterior pituitary. TSH in turn stimulates the release of the thyroxines (T_4 and the more potent T_3) from the thyroid gland. Analysis of hormone levels indicates whether there is over- or under-activity of the thyroid.

Normal range (serum values):
total thyroxine (T_4): 60–135 nmol/l
tri-iodothyronine (T_3): 1.1–2.8 nmol/l
thyroid-stimulating hormone (TSH): 0.5–5.5 mIU/l
serum free T_4: 9.4–25 pmol/l
thyroid peroxidase antibodies: $\leq$35 kU/l
serum free T_3: 3.0–8.6 pmol/l
thyroxine-binding globulin (TBG): 8–15 mg/l
T_4:TBG ratio: 6:12.

Urea and electrolytes (U&Es)

Electrolytes are minerals that are found in body tissues and blood in the form of dissolved salts. As electrically charged particles, electrolytes help to move nutrients into and waste substances out of the body's cells, maintain a healthy water balance, and help to stabilise the body's acid–base balance (pH). Electrolytes are usually determined as part of a renal profile which measures the main electrolytes in the body, namely sodium (Na^+), potassium (K^+) and creatinine and/or urea, and may occasionally include chloride (Cl^-) and/or bicarbonate (HCO_3^-) as well.

Sodium is found mainly in the extracellular fluid, outside the body's cells, where it helps to regulate the amount of water in the body. Potassium is found mainly inside the body's cells. A small but vital amount of potassium is found in the plasma (the liquid component of the blood). Monitoring the potassium concentration is important, as small changes in K$^+$ levels can affect the heart's rhythm and ability to contract. Chloride travels in and out of the cells to help to maintain electrical neutrality, and its level usually mirrors that of sodium. The main function of bicarbonate, which is excreted and reabsorbed by the kidneys, is to help to maintain a stable pH, and secondarily to help to maintain electrical neutrality.

The following values are generally accepted as the normal range, although individual values may vary slightly from one laboratory to another.

Normal range:
Na$^+$: 135–145 mmol/l, 135–145 mEq/l.
K$^+$: 3.5–5.0 mmol/l, 3.5–5.0 mEq/l.
Cl$^-$: 95–105 mmol/l, 95–105 mEq/l.
Ca^{2+} (total): 2.1–2.65 mmol/l, 8.5–10.5 mg/100 ml.
Ca$^+$ (ionised): 1–1.25 mmol/l, 4–5 mg/100 ml.
Urea: 3.0–8.8 mmol/l, 8.0–50 mg/100 ml.
Creatinine: 60–120 μmol/l, 0.7–1.4 mg/100 ml.
Bicarbonate: 24–32 mmol/l.
Lead (RBC): 0.5–1.7 μmol/l.
Cu^{2+}: 16–31 μmol/l, 110–200 μg/100 ml.
Zn^{2+}: 8–23 μmol/l, 0.05–0.15 mg/100 ml.
Mg^{2+}: 0.7 1.2 mmol/l, 1.8–2.4 mg/100 ml.
Uric acid: 0.1–0.45 mmol/l, 2–7 mg/100 ml.

Examinations

- **Bimanual examination**
- **Proctoscopy**
- **Speculum examination**

Bimanual examination

The bimanual examination is part of a full pelvic examination in which the healthcare professional inserts two fingers into the vagina and places the other hand on the abdomen so as to be able to feel the internal pelvic organs, mainly the uterus and ovaries.

The cervix is examined for size, shape and consistency as well as mobility and tenderness. While the cervix is lifted the clinician presses downward with the abdominal hand to feel the uterus (if possible). They will be examining the uterus for consistency, tenderness and size. The clinician will also feel either side of the cervix – the 'adnexal structures', notably the ovaries. Again they will be noting the size and shape of the ovaries as well as any other palpable adnexal structures.

Proctoscopy

Proctoscopy is an examination of the rectum (the final portion of the large intestine) using a metal or plastic scope called a proctoscope. The clinician gently inserts a gloved finger into the anus to check for tenderness or blockage caused by a mass lesion. The lubricated proctoscope is next carefully inserted into the rectum. It is then possible to look at the inner lining of the anus and rectum. Swabs can be taken to isolate infection, or a biopsy can be taken to look for pathology.

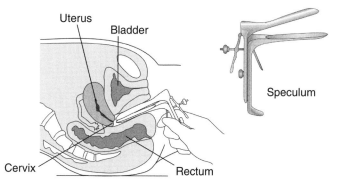

Figure 6 Speculum examination.

Speculum examination

The speculum examination is also part of the full pelvic examination process. The clinician inserts a metal or plastic speculum into the vagina. When opened, the speculum separates the walls of the vagina (which normally are closed and touching each other) so that the cervix can be seen. Thus the vagina, the vaginal walls and the cervix can be examined.

Once the speculum is in place, the clinician checks for any irritation, growth or abnormal discharge from the cervix. Certain tests can be performed by collecting cervical mucus and/or cells on a cotton swab.

Cameras

- **Colposcopy**

- **Hysteroscopy**

- **Laparoscopy**

Colposcopy

A colposcope resembles a small microscope with a light, and allows the clinician to make a more thorough examination of abnormal cells on the cervix. A liquid is dabbed on to the cervix to make the abnormal areas show up more clearly. A biopsy may then be taken from the cervix for examination under a microscope by a pathologist.

Hysteroscopy

In this technique the uterine cavity is visualised by introducing a hysteroscope (a small camera on the end of a tube) directly into the uterus via the vagina and cervix.

Laparoscopy

Laparoscopy is a surgical procedure in which a tiny flexible tube with an illumi-nated end is inserted through a small incision just below the navel. Fibreoptic fibres carry images from a lens, also located at the tip of the instrument, to a video monitor. This procedure facilitates a view of the internal abdominal and pelvic organs, as well as enabling the surgeon to take specimens for culture or micro-scopic studies if necessary.

Laparoscopy is performed in order to investigate or diagnose a range of conditions. It may be used to:

- investigate the cause of abdominal pain (e.g. a possible abscess)
- investigate the cause of gynaecological pain (e.g. endometriosis)
- investigate the cause of infertility (e.g. adhesions, scarring)
- monitor the effects of infertility drugs on the ovaries.

Laparoscopy is also used to allow viewing of surgical procedures such as:

- removal of the appendix or gall bladder
- removal of an ovarian cyst

- repair of an inguinal or femoral hernia
- sterilisation in women.

Investigations using laparoscopy are routinely performed under a general anaesthetic as day cases, without the need for an overnight stay in hospital. Laparoscopic treatment may require longer stays as an inpatient, depending on the procedure that has been performed.

A laparoscopy involves making two incisions approximately 5–10 mm long. The first incision is made just below the navel. A hollow needle is inserted, which is then connected to a supply of carbon dioxide gas, which is pumped through the needle and into the abdomen. The gas lifts the wall of the abdomen away from the internal organs, making it easier and safer to insert the laparoscope and examine the internal organs.

The laparoscope is inserted through a second small incision made in the abdomen. The exact position of the incision depends on the reason for the procedure. For instance, in women who are undergoing a gynaecological investigation, the incision will usually be made in the belly button, in order to minimise visible scarring.

If the surgeon needs to perform treatment or take samples, additional small incisions are made to allow the insertion of long thin instruments that have been specially designed for this type of surgery. At the end of the procedure, the instruments are removed, the carbon dioxide gas is allowed to escape, and the incisions are closed with stitches.

Imaging

- **Barium meal**

- **Bone density scan**

- **Computerised tomography**

- **Contrast radiography**

- **Cytometry**

- **Intravenous pyelography**

- **Magnetic resonance imaging**

- **Mammography**

- **Ultrasound scan**

- **Urodynamics**

- **X-ray**

Barium meal

This is a test in which barium (in the form of a thick white liquid formed by dissolving barium sulphate in water) is swallowed and X-rays can be used to obtain pictures of the upper gut (the oesophagus, stomach and small intestine). This is possible because X-rays do not pass through barium.

Bone density scan

In a bone scan, a radionuclide is used which accumulates in areas where there is a lot of bone activity (i.e. where bone cells are breaking down or parts of the bone are being repaired). This type of scan can therefore be used to detect areas of bone where there is cancer, infection or damage. These areas of activity are seen as 'hot spots' on the scan image. A radionuclide (sometimes called a radioisotope or isotope) is a chemical that emits a type of radioactivity known as gamma rays. A tiny amount of radionuclide is introduced into the body, usually by injection into a vein (sometimes it is breathed in or swallowed, depending on the test). Gamma rays are similar to X-rays and are detected by means of a device called a gamma camera. The gamma rays that are emitted from inside the body are detected by the gamma camera and converted into an electrical signal which is then sent to a computer. The computer builds a picture by converting the different intensities of radioactivity emitted into different colours or shades of grey. For example, areas of the target organ or tissue which emit high levels of gamma rays may be shown as red spots on the picture on the computer monitor, areas that emit low levels of gamma rays may be shown as blue spots, and various other colours may be used to show intermediate levels of gamma rays emitted.

Computerised tomography

A computerised tomography (CT) scan, also known as a computed axial tomography (CAT) scan, is a specialised X-ray test which can provide quite clear pictures of the inside of the body. In particular, it can give good pictures of 'soft' tissues of the body which do not show on ordinary X-ray pictures. The CT scanner looks like a giant thick ring. Within the wall of the scanner there is an X-ray source, and opposite the X-ray source, on the other side of the 'ring', is an X-ray detector. The patient lies on a couch which slides into the centre of the 'ring' until the part of the body to be scanned is between the X-ray source and the X-ray detector. The X-ray machine and X-ray detector both rotate around the patient's body, always remaining opposite each other. As they rotate around, the X-ray machine emits thin beams of X-rays through the patient's body, which are detected by the X-ray detector.

The X-ray detector can calculate the strength of the X-ray beam that has passed through the patient's body (the denser the tissue, the less X-rays pass through). The detector then feeds this information into a computer. Different types of tissue with different densities show up on the computer monitor as a picture with different colours or shades of grey. Thus in effect the computer creates a picture of a thin 'slice' (cross section) of the patient's body.

The couch is then moved slightly further through the 'ring' in order to obtain a picture of the next section of the patient's body. In this way several cross-sectional pictures or 'slices' of the part of the body that is being investigated are made by the computer.

Contrast radiography

A major improvement in the diagnostic accuracy of radiography has been due to the addition of contrast media which can be injected into a vein or instilled in a duct or a hollow organ (e.g. barium sulphate in the alimentary tract). A contrast medium contains relatively dense material with a high atomic number that absorbs more of the X-rays than the surrounding tissues, thus making the stomach, colon or vessel appear white on the X-ray film. It is then possible to look for structural changes such as polyps, stones or ulcerations.

Cytometry

Flow cytometry is a technique for counting, examining and sorting microscopic particles suspended in a stream of fluid. It allows simultaneous analysis of the physical and/or chemical characteristics of single cells flowing through an optical/ electronic detection apparatus. Some of the measurable parameters include the following:

- volume and morphological complexity of cells
- cell pigments
- DNA (cell cycle analysis, cell kinetics, proliferation, etc.)
- RNA
- chromosome analysis and sorting
- proteins
- cell surface antigens
- intracellular antigens (various cytokines, secondary mediators, etc.)
- nuclear antigens
- enzymatic activity
- pH, intracellular ionised calcium, magnesium, membrane potential
- membrane fluidity.

Intravenous pyelography

An intravenous pyelogram is a type of X-ray examination specifically designed to study the kidneys, bladder and ureters. After iodine-based contrast dye has been injected intravenously, a series of images are recorded at timed intervals. The kidneys are responsible for removing contrast dye from the blood and collecting it in the urine. Abnormalities in the appearance of the kidneys or ureters, distribution of contrast within a kidney, asymmetry in the amount of contrast in each kidney, or defects in the collecting systems can be identified and are suggestive of particular diseases and conditions.

Magnetic resonance imaging

Magnetic resonance imaging (MRI) is a non-invasive method of obtaining images of different parts of the body. The body can be regarded as a mass of small randomly arranged magnets. These magnets represent the nuclei of hydrogen atoms – protons – which have polarity and are thus able to alter their orientation if they are subjected to a strong magnetic field. MRI utilises these properties in a three-stage process as follows.

- **Precession.** When a patient is placed in a scanner, some of the protons within the patient become aligned along the axis of the magnetic field. When these protons become magnetised they then rotate and wobble – or precess – around the magnetised field axis.
- **Resonance.** If changes in radio frequency are then applied, the orientation of rotation and wobbling can be altered. Different types of radio-frequency pulse can be used to produce different types of emitted signal with different structures.
- **Emission.** Once the radio-frequency pulse has been turned off, the protons begin to lose their phase cohesion, and this results in the emission of very small radio-frequency signals. The magnitude, phase, amplitude and frequency of these signals are detected by a magnetic resonance imager and used to generate an image.

Mammography

Mammography is a special X-ray of the breast. It can detect most breast cancers at an early stage, before symptoms develop. All women aged 50–70 years in the UK are routinely offered a mammography every 3 years. Routine mammography is not available to women under 50 years unless they have a first-degree relative (mother or sister) who has had breast cancer at a young age. The patient's GP can advise on this.

Ultrasound scan

In ultrasound scanning a device similar to a microphone is pressed against the area to be scanned, often using some jelly to improve the contact. This device sends out very-high-frequency sound waves which pass into the area that is being examined, and bounce back when they hit an organ. This is all processed by a computer, which produces a map of the area being scanned, rather like that on a radar screen. The technique allows visualisation of static structures, and observation of moving parts (e.g. the heart of a baby in the womb, or the valves inside a heart). Most ultrasound scans are done from outside the body, through the skin, but some are done internally, using special probes (e.g. in the oesophagus to give improved views of the heart, or in the vagina to show the womb, pelvic organs and pelvic floor more clearly).

Urodynamics

Urodynamics refers to a group of diagnostic procedures that are performed in order to evaluate voiding disorders. Different tests are used for lower and upper urinary assessment.

- **Lower urinary assessment.** The most common tests are urinary flow rate and cystometry. Others include urethral pressure profile and electromyography (which assesses activity in the urethral sphincter during filling and voiding).
- **Upper urinary assessment.** Antegrade perfusion studies assess the pressure drop between the renal pelvis and the bladder. In the Whitaker test, the kidney is perfused with fluid at a constant rate of 10 ml/minute by means of a needle inserted percutaneously into the renal pelvis. A side-arm channel measures intrapelvic pressure. Intravesical pressure is measured by means of a urethral catheter.

Using the nephrostomy track, antegrade contrast studies may also be performed in order to obtain anatomical information.

X-ray

X-rays are a form of electromagnetic radiation with high energy and short wavelength, and are able to pass through body tissue. During the passage of X-rays through the body, the denser tissues, such as bone, will block more of the rays than the less dense tissues, such as lung.

A special type of photographic film is used to record X-ray images. The X-rays are converted into light, and the more energy that reaches the recording system, the darker that region of the film will be. This is why the bones on an X-ray image appear whiter (less energy passes through the tissue) than the lungs (more energy passes through).

Other tests

Heaf test

The Heaf test is a diagnostic skin test performed in order to determine whether or not a person has been exposed to tuberculosis. It is used in the UK to determine whether the BCG vaccine is needed (BCG stands for bacille Calmette-Guèrin, after the scientists who developed the vaccine). Patients who exhibit a negative reaction may be offered BCG vaccination.

The 'Heaf gun' injects purified protein derivative equivalent to 100,000 units/ml into the skin over the flexor surface of the left forearm. The test is read between 3 and 10 days later. The injection must not be administered to sites that contain superficial veins.

The reading of the Heaf test is defined by the following scale:

- negative – minute puncture scars, no induration (hardening)
- grade 1 – at least four puncture points are indurated
- grade 2 – coalescence of puncture points forming a ring of induration
- grade 3 – extensive induration (5–10 mm)
- grade 4 – severe induration ($\leq$10 mm) and possibly central blistering.

Grades 1 and 2 may be the result of previous BCG or avian tuberculosis. Children who have a grade 3 or 4 reaction require X-ray and follow-up.

Samples

- **Aspiration/biopsy**

- **Cervical smear test**

- **Chromosome analysis/karyotyping**

- **Sexual health screen**

- **Urinalysis**

Aspiration/biopsy

When a radiologist detects a suspicious area (calcifications or a non-palpable mass), or a lump has been found during a clinical or self-examination, a biopsy will be requested. A small sample of tissue is taken from the suspicious area so that a pathologist can examine the cells for signs of cancer. There are several types of biopsies (e.g. fine-needle aspiration, needle biopsy, surgical biopsy) that are performed in order to determine whether the area is benign or malignant. The results of this will guide treatment.

The testing of biopsy material for cancer involves looking at cells under a microscope for evidence that those cells have become malignant. Signs of malignancy include a change in the size of cell nuclei and evidence of increased cell division. Needle aspirations are limited in that they only show whether malignant cells are present. A tissue biopsy is needed to determine whether the cells are early-stage or invasive cancer.

Cervical smear test

This is a method of preventing cancer by detecting and treating early abnormalities which, if left untreated, could lead to the development of cancer in a woman's cervix (the neck of the womb).

The first stage in cervical screening is either a smear test or liquid-based cytology (LBC). In the former the sample of cells is 'smeared' on to a slide, which is then sent to a laboratory for examination under a microscope. LBC is a new way of preparing cervical samples for examination in the laboratory. The sample is collected in a similar way to the conventional smear, using a special device to brush cells from the neck of the womb. The head of the brush, where the cells are lodged, is either broken off into a small glass vial containing preservative fluid, or rinsed directly into the preservative fluid. The sample is then sent to the laboratory where it is centrifuged and treated to remove obscuring material (e.g. mucus or pus), and a random sample of the remaining cells is taken. A thin layer of the cells is deposited on to a slide. The slide is examined in the usual way under a microscope by a cytologist.

Chromosome analysis/karyotyping

Karyotyping is a test that is used to identify chromosome abnormalities as the cause of malformation or disease. This test can be used to:

- count the number of chromosomes
- look for structural changes in chromosomes.

The results may indicate genetic changes linked to a disease.

The test can be performed on a sample of blood, bone marrow, amniotic fluid or placental tissue. Chromosomes contain thousands of genes that are stored in DNA, the basic genetic material. The specimen is grown in tissue culture in the laboratory. The cells are then harvested, and the chromosomes are stained and viewed under a microscope. They are photographed to provide a karyotype, which shows the arrangement of the chromosomes. Certain abnormalities can be identified through the number or arrangement of the chromosomes.

Sexual health screen

This involves examination and the testing of samples to detect a range of sexually transmitted infections (STIs). A history is taken in order to identify any risk factors. The genitalia are examined for any signs of inflammation, ulceration, mites or warts, the vagina is examined for signs of inflammation, ulceration, discharge or warts, and the cervix is examined for signs of inflammation, discharge, excitation or bleeding. Vaginal swabs are taken for *Trichomonas*, bacterial vaginosis and thrush, cervical swabs are taken for gonorrhoea and *Chlamydia*, and swabs are taken from lesions for herpes (according to signs, symptoms and history). A bimanual examination detects uterine tenderness or pain, or adhesions and cervical mobility. Blood tests can detect HIV, syphilis, hepatitis and herpes.

Urinalysis

This test identifies and measures the by-products of normal and abnormal metabolism, which are eliminated from the body in the urine.

A complete urinalysis consists of three distinct testing phases:

1 visual inspection, which evaluates the urine's colour, clarity and concentration
2 chemical examination, which tests chemically for a number of substances that provide valuable information about health and disease
3 microscopic examination, which identifies and counts the type of cells, casts, crystals and other components (e.g. bacteria, mucus) that can be present in urine.

Urine for urinalysis can be collected at any time. However, the first morning sample is the most valuable one, because it is more concentrated and more likely to yield abnormal results. Because of the potential for contamination of urine with bacteria and cells from the surrounding skin, it is important to clean the genitalia first. The woman should spread the labia of the vagina and clean from front to back. The first part of the urination should be directed into the toilet, and then a sample of urine should be caught in the container provided (this is known as a midstream urine sample). Urinalysis testing is frequently carried out by dipstick testing in the clinic, in which case the results are readily available. If there is an abnormal finding, such as excessive protein or the presence of blood, it may be necessary to send the sample on to the laboratory for further analysis (microscopy, culture and sensitivities or MC&S). This will take a variable amount of time depending on the tests that need to be performed.

Useful resources

www.labtestsonline.org

McGhee M. *A Guide to Laboratory Investigations.* 4th ed. Oxford: Radcliffe Medical Press; 2003.

Contraception

- **Male condom**

- **Female condom ('Femidom')**

- **Spermicide**

- **Combined pill**

- **Patch**

- **Progestogen-only pill (POP)**

- **Injection**

- **Intrauterine device (IUD)**

- **Intrauterine system (IUS) or 'Mirena'**

- **Implant**

- **Diaphragm**

- **Emergency pill**

Hormonal and intrauterine contraception is available through dedicated community contraception and sexual health clinics, Departments of Sexual Health within hospitals (sometimes called Genito-Urinary Medicine Services) and general practice surgeries. Hormonal emergency contraception is also available from additional sources such as Accident and Emergency departments, some school nurses, and over the counter at pharmacies. Some pharmacies are involved in schemes in which hormonal emergency contraception can be obtained free of charge. Condoms are available from contraception and sexual health clinics, various commercial outlets (usually pharmacies), some bars and nightclubs, some GPs and various community schemes.

This section aims to provide an overview of the contraceptive methods that are available, describing their efficacy, how they work, and their advantages and disadvantages, contraindications and possible side-effects.

Male condom

Efficacy

The male condom is 98% effective.

How does it work?

It is put over an erect penis in order to prevent sperm from entering the vagina.

Advantages

- As well as preventing pregnancy, condoms (including the female condom) are the only contraceptive method that also protects against STIs.
- Condoms come in a variety of different types. They are available in different flavours and colours, or may be ribbed, with or without spermicide, made of latex or polyurethane, and may be sensitive or extra strong.

Disadvantages

- Condom use must be negotiated between both partners.
- The use of a condom may be perceived as interrupting sex.

Contraindications

Allergy to latex or spermicide (polyurethane condoms are available).

Possible problems

- Bursting, splitting or slipping of the condom during sexual intercourse.
- Allergy to the condom.
- Loss of sensation.

How to use a male condom[1]

Step 1	Check for (CE) mark – the European standard mark (indication of quality standard; has been tested). Check the condom is in date. Check for tears and rips in the packet. Any hole in the packet will mean the condom has dried out and may split. It is best to keep condoms in a dry, cool place. Put the condom on when the penis is erect, before there is any contact between the penis and the partner's body. Fluid released from the penis during the early stages of an erection (pre-ejaculate) can contain sperm.

Step 2	Push the condom down to the bottom of the packet and carefully tear along one side of the foil, being sure not to rip the condom inside. Teeth and nails can make a hole in the condom.
	Carefully remove the condom.
Step 3	Air trapped inside a condom can cause it to break. To avoid this, squeeze the closed end of the condom between your forefinger and thumb and place the condom over the erect penis. Be sure that the roll is on the outside.
	If you find the condom is on upside down and isn't rolling, throw it away and start again. If you just turn it around there will be sperm on the outside from the pre-ejaculate.
Step 4	While still squeezing the closed end, use your other hand to unroll the condom gently down the full length of the penis.
Step 5	Soon after ejaculation, withdraw the penis while it is still erect by holding the condom firmly in place. Remove the condom only when the penis is fully withdrawn.
	Keep both the penis and condom clear from contact with your partner's body.
Step 6	Dispose of the used condom hygienically. Wrap it in a tissue and place it in a bin. (Do not flush it down the toilet.)

Female condom ('Femidom')

Efficacy

The female condom is 95% effective.

How does it work?

Femidom is a pre-lubricated soft polyurethane sheath that lines the vagina and acts as a barrier to sperm entering the vagina. It has a smaller inner ring and a larger outer ring. The smaller inner ring is used to feed the Femidom into the vagina. Most of the Femidom goes inside the vagina, and the larger ring overlaps the outer area of the vagina.

Advantages

- The woman has control over the use of this method.
- It protects against STIs.

Disadvantages

- Some people find the female condom noisy.
- Use of the female condom may be perceived as interrupting sex.

Contraindications

Allergy to spermicide.

Possible problems

- The penis may be inserted outside the female condom.
- Some users have commented that the female condom makes a rustling noise.

How to use a female condom[2]

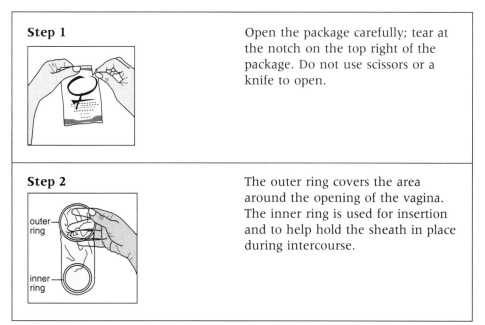

Step 1	Open the package carefully; tear at the notch on the top right of the package. Do not use scissors or a knife to open.
Step 2	The outer ring covers the area around the opening of the vagina. The inner ring is used for insertion and to help hold the sheath in place during intercourse.

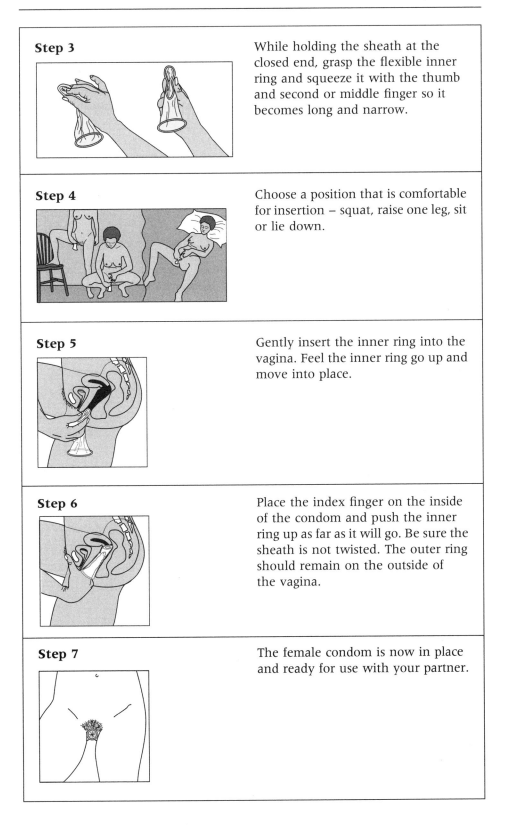

Step 3

While holding the sheath at the closed end, grasp the flexible inner ring and squeeze it with the thumb and second or middle finger so it becomes long and narrow.

Step 4

Choose a position that is comfortable for insertion – squat, raise one leg, sit or lie down.

Step 5

Gently insert the inner ring into the vagina. Feel the inner ring go up and move into place.

Step 6

Place the index finger on the inside of the condom and push the inner ring up as far as it will go. Be sure the sheath is not twisted. The outer ring should remain on the outside of the vagina.

Step 7

The female condom is now in place and ready for use with your partner.

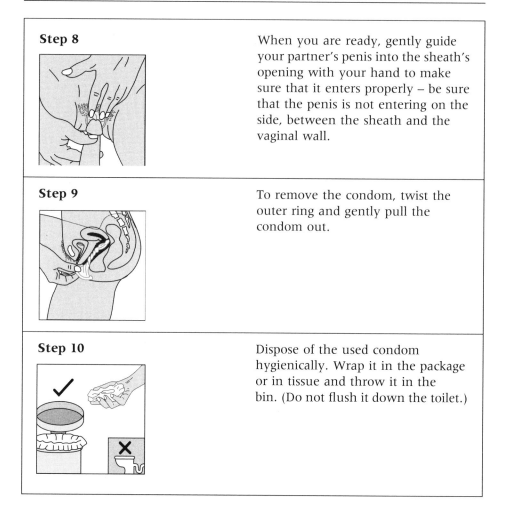

Step 8	When you are ready, gently guide your partner's penis into the sheath's opening with your hand to make sure that it enters properly – be sure that the penis is not entering on the side, between the sheath and the vaginal wall.
Step 9	To remove the condom, twist the outer ring and gently pull the condom out.
Step 10	Dispose of the used condom hygienically. Wrap it in the package or in tissue and throw it in the bin. (Do not flush it down the toilet.)

Spermicide

Efficacy

When this method is used alone its efficacy is poor.

How does it work?

It consists of a foam, cream or jelly that kills sperm.

Because it is not very effective in preventing pregnancy when used on its own, it is usually combined with another method, as a lubricant and back-up to the main barrier method (e.g. diaphragm).

Advantages

- It provides lubrication.
- Spermicide is readily available.
- It can be used with barrier methods of contraception.

Disadvantages

- Some users find it messy.
- It is not very effective when used alone.

Contraindications

Allergy to spermicide.

Side-effects

Local irritation.

Note: Condoms do not generally have spermicide on them, as there has been a reported association with increased transmission of STIs. Spermicide can irritate the epithelium and cause small cracks and cuts, which provide channels by which pathogens can enter the skin and bloodstream. The World Health Organization has recommended that condoms should have a non-spermicidal lubricant.

Combined pill

Efficacy

The combined pill is over 99% effective if taken according to instructions.

How does it work?

The combined pill contains hormones that mimic the body's natural hormones (oestrogen and progestogen). The pills stop ovulation while they are being taken. The combined pill also makes cervical mucus thicker, which prevents sperm from reaching an egg. Pills are taken for 3 weeks, and there is then a 7-day break. During this break there is usually a short, light bleed. This is not an actual period, but a 'withdrawal bleed' caused by the level of hormones dropping while the pill is not being taken. The next packet should be started on day 8, regardless of whether there is bleeding or not, in order to ensure continued protection.

This pill should be taken at the same time every day, but if forgotten can be taken up to 12 hours later. If more than 12 hours have elapsed, the pill should be taken as soon as remembered, and no extra protection is needed. If two or more pills are missed, depending on where they are in the packet, emergency contraception may be required, so consultation with a contraception specialist is recommended.

Family Planning Association
Tel: 0845 310 1334

NHS Direct
Tel: 0845 4647

If the forgotten pills are in the third week of the pack, start the next packet straight away without a break. Research has shown that after 9 days of not taking the combined pill, the ovaries can release an egg. Running on to the next packet avoids this.

Some medicines can prevent the pill from working properly. Most commonly antibiotics may interfere with the efficacy of the pill. If antibiotics are being taken, the pill should be continued, but extra precautions should be taken while the woman is on antibiotics and for 7 days after the antibiotics have finished. If the doctor prescribes any medication or if the woman obtains any herbal remedies over the counter it is important to make sure that these do not prevent the pill from working properly.

Diarrhoea and vomiting can prevent the pill from working by reducing the absorption of the pill in the gut. Extra precautions should be used while the woman is ill and for 7 days afterwards.

Advantages

- The user is in control of the method.
- There is a quick return of fertility after stopping use of the combined pill.
- It often makes bleeds lighter and less painful.
- The combined pill is protective against womb and ovarian cancer.

Disadvantages

- It needs to be taken regularly in order to be effective.
- Rare side-effects may include blood clots, increased risk of breast cancer and cervical cancer.

Contraindications

- Pregnancy.
- Breastfeeding.
- Undiagnosed vaginal or uterine bleeding.
- Past or present venous or arterial thrombosis.
- Cardiovascular and ischaemic heart disease.
- Lipid disorders.
- Focal migraines.
- Cerebral haemorrhage.
- Active liver disease.
- Oestrogen-dependent neoplasms.
- Obesity (BMI greater than $35 \, kg/m^2$).
- Severe diabetes mellitus with complications.
- Smokers over the age of 35 years.
- Family history of arterial or venous disease in a first-degree relative (mother, father or sibling) under 45 years of age.
- Acute episodes of Crohn's disease and ulcerative colitis.

Relative contraindications

- Sickle-cell disease.
- Severe depression.
- Inflammatory bowel disease in remission.
- Diseases in which high-density lipoprotein is reduced (e.g. diabetes).
- Splenectomy.
- Diseases in which drug treatment may affect the efficacy of the combined pill (e.g. tuberculosis, epilepsy).
- Diabetes mellitus.
- Obesity (BMI in the range 30–35 kg/m^2).

Possible side-effects

- Nausea (often short term).
- Breast tenderness and swelling (often short term).
- Breakthrough bleeding.
- Depression.
- Changes in libido.

A note on two specific combined oral contraceptive pills

- **Yasmin** contains the progestogen drospirenone. Drospirenone differs from other progestogens in COCs in that it has diuretic properties due to anti-mineralocorticoid activity. This may help to counteract the salt- and fluid-retaining effects of oestrogen and thus reduce fluid retention symptoms. It has also been associated in a small trial with a very small lowering of blood pressure. In addition, drospirenone is an anti-androgen, so may be an option for conditions such as PCOS.
- **Dianette** contains cyproterone acetate, an anti-androgenic progestogen, which is beneficial for women with androgenic symptoms such as hirsutism, obesity, acne, irregular periods or amenorrhoea. Dianette has an increased risk of inducing deep vein thrombosis, and is not suitable for long-term use.

Patch

Efficacy

The contraceptive patch is 99% effective.

How does it work?

The patches contain oestrogen and progestogen. These hormones are absorbed through the skin and prevent ovulation. The patch can be put on the woman's arm, thigh, back, shoulder or buttock. One patch is worn each week for 3 weeks, followed by a patch-free week.

The patch is very sticky and unlikely to become detached. However, if it does, or a new patch is not put on, advice should be sought at a clinic and condoms used until the woman is advised that it is safe to continue without a back-up method.

The manufacturer has provided the following advice.

- If the patch change day is delayed by less than 48 hours, the patch should be changed and the patch change day remains the same.
- If the patch change day is delayed by more than 48 hours, a new patch should be put on, and a new 4-week cycle begun, with a new patch change day. Extra precautions should be used for the next 7 days. A delay of 3 days or more may require emergency contraception.
- If the third patch in a cycle is left on into the patch-free week, the patch should be removed as soon as it has been remembered and a new cycle started at the normal time.
- If the patch-free interval is extended beyond 7 days, similarly to the combined pill, it is assumed that an egg may have been released after 9 days and emergency contraception is needed.

Advantages

- Some side-effects may be less than with the combined pill, as the hormones are released directly into the bloodstream.
- Only three patch changes are needed per cycle.
- The user is in control of the method.
- There is a quick return of fertility after stopping use of the pill.
- The patch often makes bleeds lighter and less painful.
- As it is similar to the combined pill, the patch may be protective against uterine and ovarian cancer.
- Daily activities such as bathing, showering, swimming and exercise can all be continued as normal without the patch coming off.

Disadvantages

- The patch needs to be changed at weekly intervals in order to be effective.
- As the hormones are similar to those in the combined pill, risks such as blood clots and cancers may be similar.

Contraindications

These are the same as for the combined oral contraceptive pill (*see* page 166).

Possible side-effects

These are the same as for the combined oral contraceptive pill (*see* page 167).
  In addition, there may be application site reactions.

Progestogen-only pill (POP)

Efficacy

The progestogen-only pill (POP) is 99% effective if taken according to the manufacturer's instructions.

How does it work?

The hormone progestogen thickens the cervical mucus, thereby preventing the sperm from reaching an egg. In some women it stops ovulation.

 The POP is taken every day without a break. It must be taken at the same time every day, and will not be effective if it is taken over 3 hours late. After this time the mucus plug at the cervix comes away and does not prevent sperm from entering the uterus. If a pill is forgotten and it is more than 3 hours late, it should be taken as soon as remembered and condoms used for the next 7 days in addition to taking the pill, until a protective level of hormone is reached.

Note: the relatively new POP Cerazette is primarily an anovulant (stops egg production), and will not be effective if it is taken over 12 hours late.

 Some drugs may interfere with the efficacy of the POP. Therefore if the doctor prescribes medication it is always best to check that it doesn't interfere with this pill.

 Vomiting within 3 hours of taking the pill may make it ineffective. Extra precautions should be taken for the following 7 days as well as taking the pill.

Advantages

- The user is in control of the method.
- There is a quick return of fertility after stopping use of the pill.
- It can be used while breastfeeding.
- It is suitable for women who are unable to use the combined pill.

Disadvantages

- It needs to be taken carefully at the same time each day.
- Periods may be irregular.

Contraindications

- Pregnancy.
- Undiagnosed bleeding from the genital tract.
- Previous or current severe arterial disease.
- Severe lipid abnormalities.
- Recent trophoblastic disease.
- Previous ectopic pregnancy.
- Current liver condition.

Possible side-effects

- Functional ovarian cysts.
- Breast tenderness.
- Feeling bloated.
- Depression.

- Fluctuations in weight.
- Nausea.
- Irregular bleeding or absence of bleeding.

Injection

Efficacy

The Depo-Provera injection is over 99% effective.

How does it work?

An injection is given once every 3 months, usually in the buttock (although it can be given in the arm or thigh). It uses one hormone, progestogen, which stops ovulation while the hormone is in the system.

Some drugs can reduce the efficacy of the injection, so it is always best to check with the doctor whether a prescribed medication will interfere with the injection.

Advantages

- Only one injection every 12 weeks is needed.
- The user is not involved (i.e. they are not responsible for the effectiveness of contraception).
- It usually stops periods. As it keeps the womb lining at the same thickness, there is no build-up of blood.

Disadvantages

- There may be some irregular bleeding or spotting initially.
- Once the hormone injection has been given it cannot be withdrawn.
- After stopping the injection it can take up to a year for ovulation to reoccur (but in some cases fertility returns as soon as an injection is due).

Contraindications

- Pregnancy.
- Undiagnosed bleeding from the genital tract.
- Previous or current severe arterial disease.
- Severe lipid abnormalities.
- Recent trophoblastic disease.
- Current liver condition.
- Severe depression.

Possible side-effects

- Headache.
- Feeling bloated.

- Depression.
- Weight gain.
- Mood swings.
- Irregular bleeding or absence of bleeding.
- Changes in libido.

Intrauterine device (IUD)

Efficacy

The IUD is 98% to over 99% effective.

How does it work?

The IUD is a small plastic T-shaped device with thin copper wire wrapped around it. It remains in the womb and is fitted by a clinician. The copper is noxious to sperm and eggs and prevents them meeting. An IUD lasts for up to 10 years (depending on the licence of the particular device), although it can be removed at any time.

The IUD is a contraceptive choice for women who have not had children. It can also be fitted as a form of emergency contraception up to 5 days after unprotected sex (or 5 days after earliest ovulation). It may be more difficult to fit an IUD in a cervix that has not been stretched through childbirth.

Advantages

- It is effective immediately.
- No hormones are involved.
- It is immediately reversible.
- The user is not involved (i.e. they are not responsible for the effectiveness of contraception).

Disadvantages

- It can make periods heavier and longer.
- It needs to be inserted and removed by a clinician.

Contraindications

- Pregnancy.
- Undiagnosed bleeding from the genital tract.
- Previous ectopic pregnancy.
- Pelvic or vaginal infection.
- Abnormalities of the uterus.
- Allergy to components of the IUD.

- Wilson's disease.
- Heavy painful periods.
- Fibroids/endometriosis.

Possible side-effects

- Heavier and more painful periods.
- Increased (but minimal) risk of ectopic pregnancy if the IUD fails.
- Wrong positioning or expulsion of the IUD.
- Pregnancy due to wrong positioning or expulsion of the IUD.

Intrauterine system (IUS) or 'Mirena'

Efficacy

The IUS is over 99% effective.

How does it work?

It is a small plastic device with a slow-release preparation of hormone in the stem. It sits in the womb, and is inserted and removed by a clinician. The hormone is progestogen, which works by thickening the cervical mucus, thereby preventing sperm from reaching an egg. It also makes the lining of the womb unfavourable for implantation. The Mirena lasts for up to 5 years. As it works in a different way to the IUD, it is not effective as emergency contraception.

Advantages

- It is effective immediately.
- The user is not involved (i.e. they are not responsible for the effectiveness of contraception).
- Periods will be much lighter, shorter and less painful.
- Periods may stop.

Disadvantages

- There may be some irregular bleeding.
- The IUS needs to be inserted and removed by a clinician.
- There is a risk of expulsion or wrong positioning.
- Pregnancy may occur if there is expulsion or wrong positioning of the IUS.

Contraindications

- Pregnancy.
- Undiagnosed bleeding from the genital tract.

- Abnormalities of the uterus.
- Uterine or cervical malignancy.
- Current liver condition.

Possible side-effects

- Breast tenderness.
- Acne.
- Headache.
- Feeling bloated.
- Mood changes.
- Nausea.
- Irregular bleeding or no bleeding.

Implant

Efficacy

- The implant is over 99% effective.

How does it work?

It is a small soft tube the size of a matchstick, and is inserted beneath the skin of the upper arm by a doctor or nurse. It is not visible but can be felt beneath the skin. Like the injection, it releases a small amount of progestogen every day and stops ovulation. It also makes the cervical mucus thicker, thus presenting a barrier that prevents sperm from reaching the egg. It lasts for 3 years.

Advantages

- It is effective immediately.
- The user is not involved (i.e. they are not responsible for the effectiveness of contraception).

Disadvantages

- The bleeding pattern can be unpredictable.
- The implant requires insertion and removal by a doctor or nurse.

Contraindications

- Pregnancy.
- Undiagnosed vaginal bleeding.
- Severe arterial disease.
- Liver adenoma.

Possible side-effects

- Irregular bleeding or no bleeding.
- Nausea.
- Vomiting.
- Headache.
- Dizziness.
- Breast discomfort.
- Depression.
- Skin disorders.
- Disturbance of appetite and/or weight changes.
- Changes in libido.

Diaphragm

Efficacy

The diaphragm is 92–96% effective if used according to the manufacturer's instructions.

How does it work?

The diaphragm is a round dome made of rubber that is used together with spermicide. It is inserted inside the vagina and covers the cervix. It provides a barrier that prevents sperm entering the cervix and reaching an egg.

Advantages

- The woman is in control of the method.
- No hormones are involved.
- It provides lubrication.

Disadvantages

- Some users find this method messy.
- The woman needs to be motivated to use it.
- The woman needs to be able to find her own cervix in order to check that the diaphragm is in the correct position.
- It is less effective than other methods.

Contraindications

Allergic reaction to spermicide.

Side-effects

- Local irritation.

How to use a diaphragm

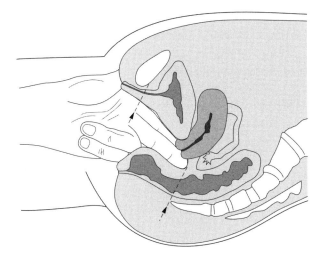

Figure 7 Diaphragm: assessing the size.

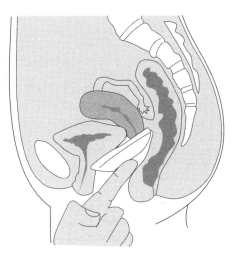

Figure 8 Checking the position of the diaphragm.

Emergency pill

Efficacy

The sooner the emergency pill is taken, the more effective it is. It can be taken up to 3 days (72 hours) after unprotected sexual intercourse.

How does it work?

The emergency pill contains the hormone progestogen. Depending on the stage in the woman's cycle at which it is taken, it either delays ovulation so that there is no egg for the sperm to fertilise or, if the egg has already been fertilised, it prevents it from implanting in the uterus.

Advantages

- It is effective in preventing pregnancy.
- The woman is in control of the method.
- It can be used after unprotected sexual intercourse.

Disadvantages

- It does not provide future contraception.
- It may disrupt the next menstrual period.
- The later it is taken, the less effective it is, and it is only 95% effective at best.

Contraindications

The effectiveness of the emergency pill can be reduced by some drugs.

Possible side-effects

- Nausea and vomiting.
- Breast tenderness.
- Headache.
- Dizziness.
- Fatigue.
- Bleeding patterns may be temporarily disturbed.

Useful resources

Faculty of Family Planning and Reproductive Health Care; www.ffprhc.org.uk
Family Planning Association; www.fpa.org.uk/guide/contracep/index.htm

References

1 www.feelconfident.co.uk/condoms/how_to_put_on_a_condom.htm
2 www.eros.shop.co.uk/how_to_use_a_femidom_guide.html

Sexually transmitted infections

- **Chlamydia**

- **Gonorrhoea**

- **Genital warts**

- **Genital herpes**

- *Trichomonas vaginalis*

- **Syphilis**

- **Thrush, bacterial vaginosis and cystitis**

- **Hepatitis**

- **Infestations**

- **HIV and AIDS**

This section covers the more common sexually transmitted infections (STIs), outlining their symptoms, how they are transmitted and the treatment available. STIs can be transmitted by penetrative sex, oral sex and digitally.

Chlamydia

Chlamydia is the commonest sexually transmitted infection in the UK. It is estimated that 10% of young people have chlamydia. Genital chlamydial infection is an important reproductive health problem, because 10–30% of infected women develop pelvic inflammatory disease (PID), which if left untreated can cause fertility problems and chronic pain.

Symptoms

The majority of women who are infected with chlamydia will have no symptoms, but some may notice the following:

- increased vaginal discharge
- frequent or painful urination
- lower abdominal pain

- pain during sex
- irregular periods.

Transmission

Chlamydia can be transmitted in the following ways:

- by penetrative sex (in which the penis enters the vagina, mouth or anus)
- from mother to baby during birth
- occasionally by transfer of the infection via the fingers from the genitals to the eyes.

Diagnosis and treatment

Samples are taken from areas that may be infected, such as the urethra and cervix in women, and are sent to a laboratory for testing. A urine sample may also be taken. The results are usually available within a week. If the test is positive, the treatment for chlamydia is a simple course of antibiotics.

Long-term effects

In women, if chlamydia is left untreated it can lead to PID, fertility problems, ectopic pregnancy and chronic pelvic pain.

Gonorrhoea

Gonorrhoea is the second commonest sexually transmitted infection in the UK. Young people are most commonly infected.

Signs and symptoms

It is possible to be infected with gonorrhoea and not have any symptoms. Symptoms can include the following:

- a change in vaginal discharge – this may increase, change to a yellow or greenish colour and become malodorous
- pain or a burning sensation when passing urine
- irritation and/or discharge from the anus.

Transmission

Gonorrhoea is most commonly transmitted via penetrative sex, and less often by the following:

- inserting the fingers in a sexual partner's infected vagina, anus or mouth and then putting them into one's own without washing one's hands in between
- sharing vibrators or other sex toys.

Diagnosis and treatment

Swab samples are taken from any area which may be infected (the cervix, urethra, anus or throat). A sample of urine may also be taken. Samples are sometimes examined immediately under a microscope, and it may be possible to make a diagnosis straight away. A second sample is sent to a laboratory for diagnosis or confirmation, and the results should be available within a week. If the test results are positive, antibiotics may be given in tablet, liquid or injection form.

Long-term effects

If left untreated, gonorrhoea can lead to PID in women. This can cause fever and pain, and can lead to scarring, causing infertility or ectopic pregnancy. A woman may pass gonorrhoea on to her baby if she is infected when the baby is born.

Genital warts

Anogenital warts (first attack) are the commonest viral STI diagnosed at genito-urinary medicine clinics. It usually takes 1 to 3 months from the time of infection for warts to appear. Not everyone who comes into contact with the virus will develop warts.

Signs and symptoms

- Pinkish-white small lumps or larger cauliflower-shaped lumps on the genital area.
- Warts on the vulva, penis, scrotum or anus, or in the vagina and on the cervix.
- The lumps may itch but are usually painless.

Transmission

Warts are spread via skin-to-skin contact and can therefore be caught as a result of any kind of genital contact as well as sexual intercourse.

Diagnosis and treatment

A clinician can usually diagnose genital warts on the basis of examination alone. A test may be performed by applying a weak vinegar-like solution to the outside of the genital area, which turns any warts white. An internal examination may be performed to check for warts in the vagina or anus.

Warts are self-limiting. However, they can be treated by freezing, burning, laser or surgical removal. There are also creams that interfere with cell reproduction or improve immunity.

Long-term effects

Some individuals will have recurrence of warts. Some types of the wart virus may be linked to changes in cervical cells that can lead to cervical cancer.

It is therefore important that all women over 20 years of age have a regular cervical smear test.

Genital herpes

Genital herpes is a virus (herpes simplex virus). Rates of diagnosis of genital herpes are highest in men and women aged 20–24 years.

Signs and symptoms

Both men and women may have one or more of the following symptoms:

- an itching or tingling sensation in the genital or anal area
- small fluid-filled blisters, which burst and leave small sores that can be painful. In time they dry out, scab over and heal. The first infection can take between 2 and 4 weeks to heal
- pain when passing urine, if it passes over any of the open sores
- a flu-like illness, backache, headache, swollen glands or fever (at this time the virus is highly infectious)
- recurrent infections are usually milder – the sores are fewer, smaller, less painful and heal more quickly.

Transmission

Herpes is transmitted via direct contact with an infected person (the virus affects the areas where it enters the body). This can be by:

- kissing (mouth to mouth)
- penetrative sex
- oral sex.

Diagnosis and treatment

- A clinical examination of the genital area is performed by a clinician.
- A sample is taken from any visible sores, using a cotton-wool swab, and sent to a laboratory for testing.

Antiviral tablets can reduce the severity of the infection, but are only effective when taken within 72 hours of the first appearance of symptoms.

During an episode of herpes, the blisters and sores are highly infectious and the virus can be passed on to others by direct contact. To prevent this from occurring, the following should be avoided:

- kissing when there are cold sores around the mouth
- oral sex when there are cold sores around the mouth, or genital sores
- any genital or anal contact, even with a condom or dental dam, when there are genital sores

- sharing towels and face flannels
- using saliva to wet contact lenses if there are cold sores around the mouth.

Long-term effects

Being infected with herpes does not affect a woman's ability to become pregnant, but if the infection occurs during the first 3 months of pregnancy there is a small risk of miscarriage. If a woman has an episode of herpes when the baby is due, she may be advised to have a Caesarean section in order to reduce the risk of infecting the baby.

Trichomonas vaginalis

Trichomonas is a flagellated protozoan. The prevalence of infection is highest in individuals aged 20–45 years.

Signs and symptoms

Often women infected with *Trichomonas vaginalis* do not have any symptoms, but discharge can occur, together with genital soreness, pain when passing urine and pain during sex.

Diagnosis and treatment

Swabs are taken from the urethra or vagina, and may be examined under the microscope and cultured. *Trichomonas vaginalis* is easily treated with antibiotics.

Long-term effects

Complications associated with *Trichomonas vaginalis* infection are rare.

Syphilis

Syphilis is a bacterial infection.

Signs and symptoms

Syphilis has three stages of symptom development:

- primary stage – sores can develop at the point where bacteria entered the body
- secondary stage – a rash can develop, warty growths may appear on the genitals, and a flu-like illness may develop
- latent stage – if left untreated, over time syphilis can lead to damage to the heart, joints and nervous system.

Transmission

Syphilis can be transmitted during the primary or secondary stages as follows:

- via oral, vaginal or anal sex
- via skin contact with any sores or rashes
- from a mother to her unborn child.

Syphilis is not usually infectious during the latent stage.

Diagnosis and treatment

A blood sample is taken together with swabs from any sores. A visual examination is performed as well as an internal physical examination for women. Syphilis is treated with a 2-week course of penicillin injections and/or antibiotic tablets or capsules. During the early infectious stages of syphillis, it is recommended that oral, vaginal or anal sex is avoided, as well as any kind of sexual activity involving contact between two people and any sores or rashes they may have, until the treatment is completed. Once the treatment has been completed they will be required to attend the clinic at regular intervals for blood tests to monitor their status.

Long-term effects

In pregnancy, syphilis can cause miscarriage or stillbirth and can be passed from the mother to the unborn child in the womb. If left untreated, syphilis can cause damage to the heart, joints and nervous system.

Thrush, bacterial vaginosis and cystitis

These conditions are not sexually transmitted. Although they can develop due to causes other than sexual intercourse, they are included here because sex can precipitate these conditions. Sexual intercourse can alter the pH of the vagina, which thrush and bacterial vaginosis may then colonise. Sexual activity can also introduce bacteria to the urethra in both men and women, causing cystitis.

Thrush

Thrush (candida) is caused by a yeast that normally lives on the skin, or in the mouth, gut and vagina, without causing any problems. Usually it is kept in check by harmless bacteria. Occasionally conditions change and the yeast multiplies rapidly, causing symptoms.

Sexual intercourse is thought to play a limited part in the epidemiology of thrush. Systemic antibiotic therapy for other conditions can cause thrush to develop, and the rise in the frequency of diagnosis could reflect increased antibiotic use as well as increased attendance at sexual health clinics.

Signs and symptoms

In women there may be one or more symptoms, including the following:

- itching, soreness and redness around the vagina, vulva or anus
- a thick, white discharge from the vagina that resembles cottage cheese and has a yeasty odour
- a swollen vulva
- pain during sex
- pain when passing urine.

The likelihood of developing thrush is increased by the following:

- wearing Lycra shorts or tight nylon clothes
- taking certain antibiotics
- using too much vaginal deodorant or perfumed bubble bath, which causes irritation
- having sex with someone who has a thrush infection
- diabetes.

Diagnosis and treatment

Thrush is diagnosed by the following:

- an examination of the genital area by a clinician
- taking swab samples from anywhere that thrush may be present, for close examination under a microscope or sending for culture.

A cream is applied to the external genital area, and women may be given pessaries to insert into the vagina using a special applicator. Oral anti-thrush tablets are also available.

Bacterial vaginosis

Bacterial vaginosis (BV) is a common infection of the vagina. It is the commonest cause of abnormal vaginal discharge in women of childbearing age, and is twice as common as vaginal candidiasis.

Although BV is predominantly a vaginal infection, there is concern that it could cause PID under certain circumstances (e.g. following surgical procedures such as termination of pregnancy, and following hysterectomy). It can cause problems in pregnancy, including late miscarriage, preterm birth, premature rupture of membranes, low birth weight, and infection after delivery. It is also thought to increase the risk of contracting HIV.

Signs and symptoms

Vaginal discharge that is whitish-grey in colour and has a fishy odour.

Diagnosis and treatment

BV is not caused by a single bacterium, but rather it is an overgrowth of various bacteria in the vagina. It is not due to poor hygiene, and in fact excessive washing of the vagina may alter the normal balance of the bacteria in the vagina, which can make BV more likely to develop. A clinician may take a vaginal swab that can be examined under the microscope, and may observe the vaginal area for discharge and a characteristic fishy odour. The pH can also be measured (BV is typically alkaline).

BV can be easily treated with antibiotics. To prevent recurrences, the following are also recommended:

- avoiding vaginal douching
- avoiding adding bath oils, detergents or bubble bath to bathwater
- not washing around the vaginal area too often.

Complications

BV during pregnancy is thought to cause some cases of early labour, miscarriage and uterine infection after childbirth. Antibiotic treatment is usually advised if BV occurs during pregnancy. If a woman has BV, the likelihood of developing a uterine infection following certain operations (e.g. termination of pregnancy) is higher. Therefore antibiotics are given before various operations of the uterus if BV is diagnosed.

Cystitis (urinary tract infection, UTI)

Vaginal intercourse has an effect on susceptibility to UTIs, although the exact mechanisms involved are still unknown. Episodes of cystitis are often associated with the onset of sexual intercourse, and women who have regular intercourse have three to four times as many episodes of infection per year as women who are not having intercourse.

Signs and symptoms

Cystitis may cause one or more of the following symptoms:

- a burning sensation in the urethra on urination – sometimes there may be blood in the urine or it may be cloudy
- the need to pass water very frequently, even when little urine is present
- a dragging ache in the lower back or abdomen.

Cystitis can be caused by any of the following:

- bacteria from the bowel
- friction during sex
- 'irritable bladder' (a particularly sensitive bladder).

Diagnosis and treatment

Over-the-counter treatments for cystitis are available. There are also several 'home remedies' that can alleviate the symptoms, including the following:

- drinking plenty of water (or any other bland liquid) to flush out bacteria and dilute the urine so that it does not sting so much during urination
- taking a teaspoonful of bicarbonate of soda mixed with half a pint of water, or any other bland liquid, every hour. This makes the urine less acidic and stops bacteria multiplying. It also eases the stinging sensation when passing urine
- taking painkillers
- some women find that drinking cranberry juice regularly can help to clear up an attack.

If the symptoms persist, the doctor will need a sample of urine in order to find out whether there is an infection for which antibiotics are required.

How to avoid cystitis

- The bottom should always be wiped from front to back.
- Drink plenty of bland fluids.
- Avoid using perfumed products on the genital area.
- Wash and pass water before and after sex.

Hepatitis

Hepatitis is inflammation of the liver. This can be caused by alcohol and some drugs, but usually it is the result of a viral infection. There are several viruses which can cause hepatitis. Both hepatitis B and hepatitis C can persist in the body and may cause chronic liver damage. Each of these viruses acts differently.

Hepatitis A

It is difficult to ascertain the prevalence of hepatitis A within the population. Cases of hepatitis A infection may not be detected through GUM clinic attendances, as individuals with such infections may not present. In addition, exposure and behavioural histories are incomplete in routine surveillance data.

Laboratory reports show that the prevalence of hepatitis A has decreased substantially over the last decade, probably due to increased awareness and vaccination. Hepatitis A diagnosis is most common in the 15–34 years age group, in which it has actually increased over the past few years. This could be attributable to increased sexual activity and world travel and lack of awareness of risk in this age group.

Transmission

- It is possible to become infected as a result of eating or drinking contaminated food or water.

- The virus is found in faeces, and can be passed on even if only a tiny amount of virus comes into contact with a person's mouth. This means that the virus can also be transmitted sexually.
- Hand-washing after going to the toilet and before eating is important.

Signs and symptoms

Individuals may have no symptoms but can still be infectious. Symptoms may include the following:

- a short flu-like illness
- fatigue
- nausea and vomiting
- diarrhoea
- loss of appetite
- weight loss
- jaundice
- itchy skin.

Diagnosis and treatment

Hepatitis A can be diagnosed by a blood test. There may be evidence of past infection which means that there has been contact with hepatitis A but there were no obvious symptoms. This may mean that there is protection from future infection with hepatitis A.

Infection is usually mild, but some people may need to be admitted to hospital.

A single injection of hepatitis A vaccine in the arm will provide protection for 1 year. A second booster injection at 6–12 months gives protection for up to 10 years. Immunisation is recommended for individuals who are travelling to parts of the world with high rates of hepatitis A. People who have been in recent contact with someone with hepatitis A may also be offered immunoglobulin in an attempt to prevent infection.

Complications

- Jaundice.
- Liver disease.

Hepatitis B

Laboratory reports show that the prevalence figures for hepatitis B have remained relatively constant over the last decade. The diagnosis is most common in the 25–34 years age group.

Transmission

The hepatitis B virus is very common worldwide. It is highly infectious and can be transmitted in a number of ways:

- via unprotected penetrative sex
- by sharing contaminated needles or other drug-injecting equipment
- by using contaminated equipment for tattooing, acupuncture or body piercing
- from an infected mother to her baby
- through blood transfusion in a country where blood is not tested for the hepatitis B virus. In the UK, all blood that is to be used for transfusion is tested.

Signs and symptoms

Some people may have no symptoms at all but can still pass on the virus. Symptoms may include the following:

- a short flu-like illness
- fatigue
- nausea and vomiting
- diarrhoea
- loss of appetite
- weight loss
- jaundice
- itchy skin.

Diagnosis and treatment

Hepatitis B can be diagnosed by a blood test. There may be evidence of past infection which means that there has been contact with hepatitis B but there were no obvious symptoms. This would give natural protection against hepatitis B. If the blood test indicates that the person is a hepatitis B carrier, this means that they can pass the condition on to others. They are also at risk of chronic liver disease, and may be referred to a specialist for further assessment. If they are diagnosed as having an active infection, they will be advised to have regular blood tests and physical check-ups. Many people do not require treatment, as inflammation of the liver may not be severe. Treatment may consist of interferon injections or antiviral tablets which can reduce hepatitis B damage.

Prevention of hepatitis B involves immunisation in injection form. Three injections of hepatitis B vaccine are given over a period of 3 to 6 months. A blood test is then performed to check that the immunisations have worked. Immunisation lasts for at least 5 years. It is important that babies of hepatitis-B-positive mothers are immunised at birth to prevent them from becoming infected.

Complications

- Jaundice.
- Liver disease.

Hepatitis C

Most hepatitis C infections occur in the 25–44 years age group. The commonest risk factor is injecting drug use, followed by receipt of blood products and transfusions. However, multiple sexual partners, sexual health clinic attendance and prostitution are also associated with an increased risk of hepatitis C infection.

Transmission

The hepatitis C virus can be spread in the following ways:

- by sharing contaminated needles or other equipment for injecting drugs
- by using non-sterile equipment for tattooing, acupuncture or body piercing
- by unprotected penetrative sex
- infected mothers may pass it on to their babies during pregnancy or at birth
- through blood transfusion in a country where blood is not tested for the hepatitis C virus. In the UK, all blood that is to be used for transfusion is tested.

Signs and symptoms

There may be no symptoms, but the virus can still be transmitted. Symptoms may include the following:

- a flu-like illness
- fatigue
- nausea and vomiting
- diarrhoea
- weight loss
- jaundice in a small number of cases
- itchy skin.

Diagnosis and treatment

Exposure to hepatitis C is diagnosed by a blood test. The first blood test will show whether an individual has ever been exposed to hepatitis C, and a further blood test is necessary to establish whether they remain infected with the virus.

Those who are currently infected with hepatitis C should be referred to a specialist for further assessment, which will include LFTs and may include a biopsy. The results of these investigations will help the specialist to decide whether treatment would be beneficial. The current medical treatment is the drug alpha-interferon. This treatment is not suitable for everyone, but some patients can be successfully treated and the drug will clear the virus.

Complications

- Jaundice.
- Chronic hepatitis.
- Cirrhosis of the liver.
- Liver cancer.

Infestations

Infestations occur where there is skin-to-skin contact, and are therefore associated with sexual intercourse.

Pubic lice

This is the crab louse (*Pthirus pubis*).

Transmission

Pubic lice are usually sexually transmitted, but may occasionally be transferred by close physical contact or by sharing bed linen or towels.

Signs and symptoms

The most common symptom is itching in the infected areas, and it may be possible to see droppings (in the form of a black powder) from the lice in underwear, as well as eggs on pubic or other hair. It is sometimes possible to see lice on the skin.

Diagnosis and treatment

The lice can be detected by physical examination and may be examined under a microscope. The infestation can be easily treated with a special shampoo or lotion. Any sexual partners of the affected person should also be treated.

Scabies

The scabies mite shows a cyclical peak in incidence roughly every 20 years in the UK, often presenting as outbreaks in schools and residential or nursing homes. Scabies is more prevalent in urban than in rural areas, and in winter than in summer. It is more prevalent in children and young adults, but all age groups can be affected.

Transmission

Scabies is not necessarily sexually transmitted, as any close physical contact can spread the infection.

Signs and symptoms

The main symptom of scabies is an itchy rash on the hands, wrists and elbows, underneath the arms, and on the abdomen, breasts, genitals and buttocks.

Diagnosis and treatment

The rash can be seen on physical examination and may be examined under a microscope. Scabies can be easily treated with a special shampoo or lotion.

HIV and AIDS

Human immunodeficiency virus (HIV) attacks the body's immune system, impairing its ability to fight off infections. It targets specific white blood cells known as CD4 cells. The lower a person's CD4 count, the weaker their immune system will be. The number of AIDS diagnoses and deaths in HIV-infected individuals declined after the introduction of effective therapies in the mid-1990s, and in more recent years the figures have remained relatively constant. Sex between men and women overtook sex between men as the most common route of HIV transmission in 1999.

Transmission

HIV is transmitted via the body fluids or blood of an infected person. This usually happens as a result of sexual intercourse with an infected person or sharing needles with an infected person. Mothers may pass on HIV to a child at birth (HIV can also be transmitted in breast milk), and a very small number of people become infected as a result of receiving infected blood transfusions. Oral sex carries some risk of infection, as infected fluid could get into the mouth, where the virus could enter the bloodstream via bleeding gums or sores. Infection resulting from oral sex alone is very rare.

Signs and symptoms

- No early symptoms.
- Flu-like symptoms.
- Fever.
- Headache.
- Tiredness.
- Enlarged lymph nodes.

Diagnosis and treatment

HIV is detected by means of a blood test. Individuals who may be infected are advised to wait for 3 months after the last risky sexual contact before having the test. This is because the virus is not detectable during this initial 'window period.'

Useful resources

British Association for Sexual Health and HIV (BASHH)

Website: www.bashh.org
The British Association for Sexual Health and HIV was formed in 2003 through the merger of the Medical Society for the Study of Venereal Diseases (MSSVD) (established in 1922) and the Association for Genito-Urinary Medicine (AGUM) (established in 1992). It provides information on the latest developments, clinical guidelines, conferences and courses.

Society of Health Advisers in Sexually Transmitted Diseases

Website: www.shastd.org.uk
This organisation provides answers to frequently asked questions about STIs, information about infections and treatments, a discussion forum and details of GUM clinics around the UK.

Sexually Transmitted Infections (STIs)

Website: www.nhsdirect.nhs.uk/SelfHelp/info/advice/stis.stm

This website provides a straightforward but brief outline of sexually transmitted infections (STIs) and their treatment. It is part of the NHS Direct website.

Index